The Master's Manual

The Master's Manual

A Handbook of Erotic Dominance

Jack Rinella

Edited by Joseph Bean

Daedalus Publishing Company
584 Castro Street, Suite 518
San Francisco, CA 94114 USA

Published by Daedalus Publishing Company, 584 Castro Street, Suite 518, San Francisco, CA 94114 USA.

Cover design by Don Mooring

ISBN 1-881943-03-8

Library of Congress Catalog Card Number: 93-74629

Printed in the United States of America

To Tom Brennan, whom I love very much
and who's always been willing to listen.

TABLE OF CONTENTS

Chapter

EDITOR'S NOTE

Editing this book has not been a grand give and take or a battle between the author and the beast (editor) as work on first books often is. It has been no battle at all. The author has presented his ideas and opinions honestly and in unambiguous language. My job has been to dot Is and cross Ts so that the author's thinking is conveyed to you clearly and without distraction. That, in and of itself, can be a tedious job, but not with this subject matter.

I am glad I undertook the editing of *The Master's Manual*. Reading Jack Rinella this closely has been a learning experience, a thought-provoking and engaging challenge. Like any text on a subject so likely to be controversial, this book is a very personal document. The sense and substance of every one of these 40 pieces is— unless I have erred in judgement or understanding—still entirely Jack's. His book bundles up his thinking and realistically reflects his mind. It proves that his is one of the voices we ought to hear in the on-going conversation in which we, the active leatherfolk of the 1990s, are working out our self-definitions, mapping out the territories of our lives, and staking out the frontiers of desire and experience we intend to explore.

The Masters Manual stands as a significant contribution to the process of recording and determining who we are and what we are becoming. Any participation in that process—even one as slight as adjusting Rinella's punctuation—is valuable, and gives the participant a certain sense of fulfillment. Here, says the effect, you were a cog or a gear in the great machinery of becoming which is manufacturing self esteem, self expression, and self realization for an under-encouraged community.

Thank you, Jack, for your friendship and for trusting me with your brainchild.

Joseph W. Bean, San Francisco, October 1993

Chapter 1

AN INTRODUCTION

Matt's friend, JR, invited him to come to my annual International Mr. Leather open house. So it was actually in my own apartment that I first met him. He was attractive, 5'11", a hunky 26 year-old with a closely trimmed beard and a bright, appealing smile. I liked him immediately, as I do most men his age.

In the course of the next few days, I got to know him and his dream: he wanted to be a master.

The fact that he was brand new to leather and didn't know very much about it prompted him to ask that I teach him. He'd read my weekly columns in Gay Chicago Magazine for almost a year and felt that I could give him the start in leather that he needed. Far be it from me to pass up an opportunity like that.

I became his mentor. I went to my computer and printed out the seven or so columns that I knew held ideas about being a master. And that's how this book was born.

It goes back a bit earlier than that, actually. The essays in this book were written because I was in the right place at the right time. One Friday afternoon I overheard Ralph Paul Gernhardt, Publisher of Gay Chicago Magazine, talking about his desire to find someone to write a weekly column about leather. I volunteered to bring in some writing samples. A week later he hired me.

It was really an improbable scenario. I was relatively

new to Chicago, an unknown leatherman, never before published in the gay press, and here I was with a weekly readership of over 20,000 people, all expecting me to be an expert on leather and SM.

My leather encounters began over a decade ago, again because I was in the right place at the right time.

I was cruising the halls of a bath house in Philadelphia when I noticed this handsome young man sitting in a cubicle. We talked and he asked me to help him celebrate his birthday. He had brought along several lengths of rope, and wanted someone to tie him up for his birthday. I did, and the rest is history.

From that history—a life lived in the Midwest with frequent visits to the major leather cities of America—I gained the experience that made me the leatherman I am today. This book is the result of reading, playing, and thinking a lot about SM.

In these pages you're going to find practical advice, "do-able" suggestions, true stories of SM encounters, a bit of eroticism, and my own philosophy on SM. All of that should be helpful, but none of it will make you a leather master or mistress. You need more than that.

One thing you need is to believe in yourself. As you learn, grow, and experience leathersex, you'll decide that you know what you're doing, and you'll want to take more control of the situation. As you become more and more successful at doing just that, you'll be more and more a master.

There are two qualities that make a leatherman: proper technique and the right attitude. Attributes such as physique, education, personality, charisma, and "who you know" certainly help, but they are superficial to the real master's persona. The kind of people who stand out as masters know what to do, and they *know* that they know what to do.

They have the skills needed to tie safe knots or swing a good whip. They have the self-confidence necessary to discipline themselves and others. They've found men and women to play with and have grown through their experiences. They accept the responsibility to be safe, sane, and consensual while never (or almost never) forgetting to have fun.

Pleasure is the rhyme and reason for leather. To be even more clear, it is the reason for leathersex.

Not every leather encounter ends in an orgasm, nor even becomes a sexual event. But, by and large, what I'm talking about, and what I practice, is human sexual activity with a "spicy" flavor. It's sex with toys and bondage and pain and domination and submission. It's not all those things all the time, but it's enough of those things enough of the time that leather is my lifestyle.

Many of the chapters in *The Master's Manual* were first published separately, and each can be read out of context. But the real message of these pieces can only be discovered when they're all taken together.

Being a master is not just one thing, or two or three things, but a mindset and lifestyle with many aspects, some overlapping, some more important than others. A mosaic is made up of many pieces. Individually, the parts don't make sense until you step back and see them in relationship to each other. Similarly, mastery doesn't make sense, until you have the perspective to see it for what it really is: not necessarily one activity or another, but rather a whole way to relate, to be true to yourself while allowing the others in the "scene" to be themselves as well.

There are no secrets in this book. SM, whether

practiced as a master, a slave, a top or a bottom, is nothing more than another way for humans to relate. SM needs the same interpersonal skills, the same common sense, and the same desire for experience that any human endeavor demands.

On the surface SM may seem extravagant, intense, even extreme. In reality it's only people being people. The best SM, of course, is real people being real. The "reality" of their SM scene may be fleeting, may be playful, and may even be preposterous, but it is what they have chosen for that moment.

Live fully in those moments, and in every other moment, for life is what we have and, in fact, it is probably the only thing worth having.

Before you plunge into the next pages, I'd like to take care of two pieces of business.

First, SM is no place (in fact there is NO place) for racism, sexism, ageism, or classism. I have tried to keep my pronouns reflective of the fact that SM is for males and females and those who defy gender categorization. Therefore, I sometimes write "he or she", sometimes "they", sometimes "master" or "mistress." All the gender-bending semantics can get burdensome, so please bear with me. I mean to include all of you, as you are, and if sometimes I sound a little too male, forgive me, but that's me.

My last therapist assured me I was well-adjusted. As such I am a happy gay male. But SM knows no restrictions as to race, creed, color, ethnic origins, or sexual orientation. Enjoy it, whoever you are.

And secondly, I have to acknowledge my deep

indebtedness to the men and women who gave me the wonderful life experiences that empowered me to become an author. You are all too numerous to list: Joe, Rose Marie, Michael, Andrea, Lorin, my grandmothers, and the rest of my biological family, even if you never see this book!

Lynn, who is so much the ideal leather master.

My lovers and exes, my friends, my fuck-buddies, my boys, et al: Steven L., Jim D., Bart M., Ann C., Richard S., David M., Keith M., Larry P., Tom S., Tom B., Rick R., Rick A. and Dean H., Gary M., John B., Donn F., Donna G., Maria V., John N., Lee M., Vinnie D., Paul V., and Dick M.

Ralph G., and Jerry W. from Gay Chicago Magazine who gave me the break I needed, and Karen R., as well.

My teachers, especially Henry F., Sister Mary Carmel, and Brother Joseph.

And those who've passed on: Robert R., Don F., Gary A., Michael H., Patrick B., Richard L., and David H.

Thanks to each of you, and to all the other unsung heroes in my life as well.

Jack Rinella

Chapter 2

WHAT IS LEATHER?

Leather bars have changed. You'll hear lots of stories about bars from the 60s and 70s that have long since passed into history. In the 90s, the only ball action on the top of the pool table is with wooden spheres. Dress codes are less stringent. Real masters are hard to find, "wanna-be's" circulate hopelessly for hours, and eventually settle for quick anonymous action.

Time was when a good leather bar had water sports, public sex, significant areas for bondage and whipping, and back rooms that started at the coat check area. And most guys checked a lot more than their coats!

Things have changed. These are the 90s and we have both the plague of AIDS and a significant right-wing monitoring of public areas, especially bars. Bar owners and patrons may long for the good old days, but we know that to allow such activity would be to invite immediate revocation of liquor licenses.

One might ask if there are any leather bars left? But in reality there is a more fundamental question: "What is leather?"

I know a few guys who are into leather *as leather*. They enjoy the feel of the material. They find its smell erotic. Many love the sound of leather rubbing on leather. A few of these leather aficionados are so focussed on their leather fetish that they never venture into the *other* world of leather. By that I mean that sado-masochism and its related activities such as bondage, discipline, verbal abuse, and the like are not a part of every leather lifestyle. On the other hand, for those who enjoy an intense master/slave relationship such a leather *as leather* scene leaves a lot to be desired.

Leather is a state of mind, an attitude, a mode of perception. We of the leather community share beliefs about power, lifestyle, experience, and world view.

Power. We incorporate power as a recognizable aspect of our lives. We use it for our own ends, whether in domination or submission. Either way we employ its effects for our own pleasure, experience and growth. We do not shun power, but include it as an active part of our lifestyle. For that reason, roles such as master and slave have meaning, as do the authority figures represented by uniforms, and the strength portrayed by levis, chains, and arm bands.

Lifestyle. We choose lifestyles that reflect our inner feelings. We seek others to share that lifestyle with us in social, sexual, and political ways. We live lives that afford us the ability to share power in some form. This may be as casual and fleeting as a back-room trick or as encompassing as a formal, long term, live-in daddy/son relationship.

Experience. Experience is the glue that brings and keeps us together. There is a significant amount of bonding in clubs, in sexual role play, in common attire and space. Without a partner, much leather activity would be impossible. We need each other in order to create the experience. We need the milieu in order to explore its richness. It is the activity—not the discussion of it—that is the essential foundation of the leather life.

Eventually, of course, we internalize all this as a *world view* that gives cohesiveness to leather. The framework can be seen delineated in club rules, dress codes, leather writings and videos. John Preston's *Mr. Benson*, Larry Townsend's *Leatherman's Handbook*, the magazines *Manifest Reader* and *Drummer* are but a few of the media that give voice to this structure.

All of this is merely ephemeral until it is lived in a practical way. Leather is more than a philosophical outlook. It is a way of acting and living. It is the clothes we wear, the sexual activities we pursue, the tribes we create, the spaces we enjoy. It is most of all the decisions we make: to live by the drummer in our own hearts, seeking a powerful, sensuous, open, and truthful life.

We fall short of these goals. But we pursue them nonetheless.

For me, leather is the recognition of the strength of the god-man I am, and a desire to bond with him in the others I meet. For me it is sado-masochism, manly strength, and sweaty bodies. It is bonding in domination and submission, the enjoyment of pain and the sharing of pleasure. It is the squeak of black leather jackets rubbing in the dark, the heat of impassioned bodies, and the assurance of spoken affirmations.

What is leather? It's all those things. Leather is a "head-space" that allows these dreams to take shape. It is a meeting of kindred spirits, from which I embark on the search for the satisfaction of my quest. What will I find? The man I want to be and the men with whom I want to share that being.

Chapter 3

THE MAKING OF A MASTER

From birth we are socialized to be conforming, compliant, and behaved—that is, to act like bottoms. Conformity to society's standards is the requirement for acceptable behavior, and we are consistently and constantly reminded of that fact. We don't all do so, but socialization is still the rule proven by few exceptions.

The rare breed of person who hears a different drummer and is willing to choose a lifestyle not acceptable to mainstream America does exist. Specifically of course, leatherfolk live that kind of lifestyle. Whether one chooses a role as top or bottom, we are outside the acceptable limits of human behavior.

Paradoxically, leather masters, so very non-conforming as regards sexual behavior, are also the heroes, the models, and the idols. In a sense, they are the Lone Rangers, the explorers, the conquerors, and the self-made men and or women. I've never said that our society is consistent—it just wants its members to be that way.

Since leather mastery is counter-cultural, the quick and easy way to become the real master, which so many wish for, does not exist. Experience is still the best teacher. And what does experience teach?

Reflecting on the masters I admire, I notice several traits they have in common. They have learned technique, self-confidence, consistency, reliability, self-awareness, care,

21

and patience. Yet, their approaches vary. Some focus more on one aspect of SM than another. Each has his or her own degree (and form) of sadism, finds enjoyment in varying intensities of sexual gratification, has a unique personal belief system, and defines the service they wish to receive in a very personal way.

But how do they get that way? To say "by experience" lacks any kind of practical meaning. Let me therefore add some detail.

1. They find other masters and submit to them.

Most of them have experienced some kind of domination from another. That may not mean that they have been "slaves" or even bottoms. What it means is that they have put themselves into positions where they could find out what those who submit to them would feel.

They've allowed themselves to be bound, disciplined, pinched, poked, and generally dominated. Invariably they did it for the experience.

A master/friend of mine once showed me a new pair of tit clamps that he had bought. They were simply four prongs that had a rubber ring to tighten them. They looked like they would hurt.

His first comment was that they hurt. How did he know? Like most conscientious tops he had tried them on himself first.

2. They do their homework.

Trying something out on yourself first is "doing homework." Additionally, though, real masters get that way by finding out whatever they need to know about SM. Invariably, they have read a lot of books and magazine articles, attended workshops and demonstrations, and taken the extra effort needed to become proficient in leather.

You can certainly have a good time in leather on a catch

as catch can basis, but as in anything else, real mastery takes a commitment of time, energy, money, and desire. Half-assed, half-hearted involvement will show.

3. They are mature through self-knowledge and raised consciousness.

Until you are willing to deal with your own inner issues, your emotional barriers, and your pre-conceived ideas, you will never be able to realize the real you. If you lead your life kidding yourself, suppressing your feelings, and avoiding the truth, that is the kind of leather life you are going to live.

Find ways to understand yourself, and you will be able to become the person of your fantasies. For fantasies to become real, real people must accept them, create them, and experience them. Otherwise we are only talking about fantasies that will never come to fruition.

4. They are self-controlled.

Mastery of another is a steady process that takes time, insight, and decisive behavior. Many factors have to be weighed and acted upon. The real master is in control of himself and his feelings so that all of his being can be orchestrated toward his goal of domination.

There is a great temptation, of course, to let things slide in a master/slave relationship, to let the goal of mastery slip by under the sway of pleasure, frustration, weariness, or emotion. If you can't control yourself, you will never really control another.

5. They have reflected on who they are and what they want.

I may be repeating myself here. This is more of the idea of self-confidence and self-knowledge. But I repeat it in order to underscore that real masters accept that they are masters. They will acknowledge their desire to dominate and control. They admit that they are sadists. They embrace their own selfishness. They are willing and able to be served, worshipped, and waited upon without regret or guilt.

6. They have actively sought to become better masters.

Luck does not make masters. People become masters by their own decision to embrace that lifestyle and to allow themselves to change into the kind of master they wish to be. It's not by mistake that masters rule, but because of specific actions they have taken to achieve their very purposeful goals.

7. They seek persons over whom they can exercise their mastery.

Masters and slaves go together. You can't be one without having the other. In order to leave the realm of the wanna-be's you have to find your fantasy's complement.

Take it from me: finding that master or slave is not easy. Real masters have become such because they searched to find the men and women who would be their slaves. Potential slaves are out there, but you must work to find them and work to earn their enduring service.

8. They have mentors.

No one gets where they are going by themselves. Likewise, those who want to be masters seek out those who can teach them by discussion, by example, by experience.

Sometimes this mentoring is mutual, sometimes it is from a slave, often it is short-lived. The ideal, of course, is to find a master you can respect and ask him or her to mentor you. Be willing to submit to his or her instruction. Become a student and learn by listening and obeying.

The time will soon come when you will out-grow the mentor, but the lessons, and the speed of the learning, will have made it worthwhile.

Chapter 4

WHAT WE REALLY NEED
IS AN EDUCATION

Over the years, several men have come to me with the request: "Will you teach me to be a better top?" Many more have asked the similar question, "Will you help me become a really good slave?" Though I'm never reluctant to try, doing either of these things can be a difficult and time-consuming endeavor. Of course, the effort has its own rewards. The pleasure of leathersex is undeniable. It seldom fails to satisfy the hedonist in me.

The teacher in me strives to reach high standards, to bring out the best in each person's potential. That can be a difficult task. Successful training is dependent on a great many variables outside the instructor's control. Real learning requires the willingness to question the status quo, to accept reasonable (and sometimes unpleasant) conclusions, and then to make the changes necessary to achieve your goals.

It would be fun to have an SM Academy. Just interviewing prospective students would be an incredible thrill. Can you see it now? Each applicant would fill out a questionnaire, send photos, and describe his/her aspirations. We could pair tops and bottoms in the same class. Laboratory workshops would be conducted. Why, I bet no one would ever cut class!

Describing how I learned to be a master is a long story

and I'm not sure anyone would believe it. But the short telling of it is simple: Practice, practice, practice. Over the years, willing partners demonstrated techniques, loaned me equipment, suggested various activities, and most importantly, allowed me to try things out. Interspersed, there was a good deal of reading on the subject, and significant thought and discussion. SM is not a mindless or thoughtless activity. If we mistakenly approach it that way, we open ourselves up to the less appealing, and even dangerous, aspects of leather. Leather is a full exploration of one's humanity: physical, mental, emotional, sexual, social, and spiritual.

Admittedly, the word "training" is often applied to a leather scene that has absolutely no educational value. Most scenes are conducted for the pleasure of the sado-masochism and the joy of the orgasm—which is fine. Experiences need not be continually wrapped in deep meaning and serious personal exploration. Just do it for the fun of it.

On the other hand, the development of good technique and the personal growth of the participants demand that time be spent in learning the ropes. Such instruction would cover three areas: technique, understanding, and attitude.

Technique is the easiest to learn. Many clubs provide lectures and workshops where technique is demonstrated and shared.

Understanding comes from discussion, reading, and reflecting about one's experiences. It seeks to satisfy the question "Why?" That is a very important activity. Why we do what we do is critical. Sadomasochistic play is no place to express anger, fear, or self-aggrandizement. If you don't know why you're letting yourself be beaten or why you are the one inflicting the pain, then you'd better find out before you continue your "games."

Finding out is a life long process. The value of wisdom ought never be ignored.

Successful SM is critically dependent upon the right mindset. We'll be quick to agree that bottoms and slaves need the right attitude, but more importantly, those in control, or who profess to be in control, need sensitivity, tolerance, self-confidence, compassion, and intuitive perception. Gaining these, you gain a rich and enormously valuable ability to live your fantasy life.

How do we learn these things? I've never seen them listed in the curriculum of any school I've ever attended! We learn them by experimentation with competent mentors, by our willingness to change as we discover our inner selves, and by gaining wisdom in the various ways it tries to come to us.

Myriad ways to learn are presented to us on a daily basis. Our own willingness to learn will allow them to affect us in positive ways. More importantly, we need to have the attitude of a student. In my experience, that means asking questions. The only "dumb question" is the one not asked: the unasked question goes unanswered, leaving us unchanged and uneducated.

It's not always easy to phrase a question or to speak it out loud. Sometimes, to do so takes courage. I always suggest it's best to ask it poorly, with the chance then to re-phrase it properly, than not to ask it at all.

There's a lot to learn about SM, and knowing its techniques and purposes unfolds a rich and rewarding vision of possibilities and pleasures. So don't be afraid if you have a lot to learn, there's a lot worth learning, just waiting for you to ask.

Chapter 5

REFLECTIONS ON A SCENE

Every scene is the unique creation of the men and women in it, as influenced by time and space.

He had me report at 10 am on Saturday, wearing a tee shirt, jeans, and sneakers. I got there ten minutes early. "Sir, i hope you don't mind i'm early."

"We'll see about that, boy. Come in," he said.

I followed him into the library. He was a handsome blond, trim for his age. He sat on the couch. I stood apprehensively. This was my first time with him. He asked me a few questions about safe sex practices, any limits I might have, and whether I needed a safe word or cue to end a scene. I said I didn't.

"Strip then, boy," he ordered. I did, and he motioned for me to follow him.

We went into his basement. He lit a few candles, turned down the lights. "Nice body for a man my age," he said. Ironically, I was the same age as my master. He rubbed his hands over me, inspecting and caressing my hairy chest and ass. He put a collar around my neck, then attached wrist restraints.

He positioned me under some eye hooks in the rafters and clamped me in place. It had been a long time since I had gone bottom for a man.

I was hanging there, legs dutifully spread as he commanded, arms raised high. First one tit and then the other was clamped, then a hood blinded me. As he continued, I counted as he attached 25 clothespins to my skin. I had to use my breathing exercises to relax and lessen the pain. There was no sense in resisting the pain, I knew. If I could flow into it, my body's hormones would take over sooner and the pain would lessen.

He didn't keep the clothespins on me very long, and as he removed each one, he rubbed the sore spot as if to make the pain go away. Then he released my bonds and pushed me to my knees.

"Clean my boots," he said. I licked the black leather. His boots were clean. I loved the smell and the feeling of the hard leather. I moved into a subservient role. It was peaceful. I asked to lick the soles of his boots. He lifted his foot.

When he was satisfied, he pressed my face into the jeans covering his crotch. He was erect. I wanted to mouth his prick.

Instead he clamped me back into a spread eagle position, and I heard him leave the room. In a matter of minutes he returned. Soon I heard an electric clipper. I smiled to think what my lover would say when I came home smooth.

I felt the vibrations on my butt, my back, my abdomen. Then he applied water and shaving cream . . .

A scene is filled with variation. To think that what you've just read is how it will be isn't very realistic. What makes a scene is really *who* makes the scene. Every top is different and most tops are different with different bottoms.

There was very little verbal communication between my master and me. On the other hand, when I'm master I ask a lot of questions, using words to reinforce my slave's submission. I'm not very good at verbal abuse; others make it their specialty.

Some scenes start in a bar, two strangers getting to know each other, testing and probing to find if this top is the one with the technique or if this bottom has the right stuff. Many men who have "played" have met first via letters, phone conversations, or e-mail on one of the many gay computer bulletin boards.

When he had me smoothed to his liking, he took a break, offered me a beer, and told me to sit on the floor. It was a breathing spell. He told me to look at my stomach. It hadn't been that pale, that denuded in years. In due time he took me over his knee, spanking me with his bare hand. He started slowly at first, allowing my ass to get used to his strokes.

In no time at all I was back "in position." He took a cat-o-nine tails off the wall and proceeded to give color to my back. He never hurt me, but he let me feel his dominance.

I always tell my bottoms that I won't hurt them, but I will give them pain. And, indeed, none have ever been hurt. Black and blue maybe, but never hurt. The pain is only an entry-way into a euphoric space.

He stopped the beating and gently caressed my reddened skin. I could feel my senses drift. I experienced a sense of freedom, even as the wrist restraints kept me in place.

He stood behind me, rubbing his crotch into the cleft of my naked ass, hugging me and playing with my tits. Strong feelings surged through me. I could love this man. I did love this man. I wanted to belong to this man.

Not every session is as good as this one. Not every master as expert, nor every slave as practiced.

But when you find the partner you can trust, the one who is able to fathom your fantasies, leathersex becomes a special act, one I doubt I'll ever fully describe in these pages.

May you find a master as fine as you wish, a bottom as fine as you deserve.

Chapter 6

WHY SM?

There are probably as many reasons for enjoying SM as there are people who practice it. My comments, in answer to questions as to why we leathermen "do those things," merely reflect my experiences and feelings. I'm not pretending to speak for all the leather community.

My viewpoint, for the most part, is that of a sadist and master. Simply put, I enjoy taking control and giving my partner the physical, mental, emotional, and spiritual experiences he desires.

The SM that we leathermen practice is consensual and sane. It is pain without violence, humiliation without degradation, and bondage without victimization. If you don't believe me, then you have not experienced the joy of SM that we who approach it that way know so well.

The strongest attraction that leathersex holds for me is the bonding that I experience in the activity. It is a bonding that lasts and grows. In a real sense my slave and I become one in a tapestry, the event of the submission/domination which we create. It is a mutual event. In every sense, as I make him my slave, he actively and completely makes me his master. It is a complimentary and fulfilling event. My mastery is just as much his creation as his slavery is mine.

Secondly, the real "event" of SM is the transition into an altered state. As paradoxical as it may seem, bondage gives one a sense of freedom; physical stress, a feeling of relief. The pain creates (biologically and otherwise) a strong feeling of pleasure. (Refer to *Urban Aboriginals* by Geoff Mains for a fuller treatment of this phenomenon.)

The deepest and best SM experiences reveal a spiritual universe of immense proportions. The participants find themselves adrift in an ecstatic sea of color, depth, music, expanse, and love. That is not to say every experience develops this way. All that can be said is that every experience is the unique creation of the men and women who are in the leathersex relationship at the time.

For each of us that means something different. Some get off on the pain of spanking, others enjoy the loss of power, the shedding of "everyday roles." Some seek sons, others daddies. I've lost count of the men I've had leathersex with, but what does remain is the memory of unique, giving, seeking, and passionate brothers who trusted me and taught me as they opened themselves to me. They shared their souls with me and in that way my soul grew as well.

Not everyone into leather is into SM. Some glory in the feel, smell, and sound of cowhide; others prefer mutual, peer-to-peer scenes. Many avoid activities that cause pain. What is common is the shift into a different, and very personal world-view. What is universal is the permission to live one's dreams.

Some are able to allow themselves to live their dreams full-time and to live the lifestyle wherever they go. For others, it is an occasional diversion from everyday reality. What is consistent is the assertion of self that one makes when one becomes what one wants to be. A vest and its badges may bring stares. The chain around a bottom's neck may draw ridicule. What is significant here is not the reaction of those looking on, but the intention of those who are stating and living their preferences. They are men and women with the courage to live their dreams. They are people willing to show that reality is created by our choices, and to demonstrate that we choose the experiences we wish.

Why SM? For me it is the truth of who I am . . . and for us in leather that is the answer that matters.

Chapter 7

THE GOALS OF LEATHERSEX

There's a garbage dumpster down the street covered with an old, worn poster that urges everyone that passes by to "Destroy Power." It's what's left of some radicals' "Dump Bush" campaign. I pass by it frequently, and it invariably makes me think about the use and abuse of power.

So I was going to write in this chapter about power and leather, about the neutrality of power, and its necessity and inevitability in our lives. I would have discussed the concept of empowerment as a goal of good SM.

As I was contemplating that topic though, I realized that empowerment is only one of the goals of SM, and that ecstasy and bonding are equally important, and as often sought.

It's not as if we go into a leather bar or read the classifieds looking for someone to bring us to ecstacy or empower our lives. We probably don't even think about looking to bond with Ms. or Mr. Right. No, our minds are much more focussed on the pursuit of pleasure, the fulfillment of lust, looking to pass the night, meet friends, or satisfy curiosity.

Once again, I'd like to stress that "We do it for the fun of it." Plain and simple, SM is fun, perhaps serious fun, but fun nonetheless. That truth having been emphasized, let me talk about the three elements that make it fun.

1. Empowerment

Appearances are deceptive. The bottom that hangs there, blindfolded, cuffed and roped spread eagle, with clothespins on his tits, perhaps his ball sack stretched and weighted, looks helpless. And I'm sure that that is physically so.

In a scene like that, it is easy to say that the top has assumed a powerful position, and indeed feels empowered by his domination of a hapless "victim." But that's only a small part of what's going on.

In the first place, in safe, sane, and consensual leather SM there are no victims. The one bound is consenting, and remains in power insofar as his (or her) consent is absolutely necessary for the scene to continue. By accepting the dominant role, the top has agreed to be responsible. The bottom's health and welfare depend upon it.

I have hung there "helpless." It is one of the prerequisites for incredible feelings. Because I have experienced the bondage, the pain, and the helplessness, I have become empowered. I have faced the fear and the anguish, and survived. In passing through this proverbial "fire," I have become stronger, more self-aware, more sure of my ability, myself. I passed the test and the passing empowered me in the scene and afterwards.

2. Ecstacy

More and more often, the SM experience is discussed in terms of ritual, alternate spaces, religious awakening, and bliss. How and why those spiritual events happen, and even how often they happen, remains a mystery.

It's not always easy to get leatherfolk to share their very personal experiences in this realm. Language fails in describing what transpires, but over and over again, once we get past the vagueness of words, leatherfolk admit to the experience of psychic, religious, and extra-sensory phenomena.

To make ecstacy the center of SM is misleading. As far as I can tell, such experience is rare, fleeting, and often surprising, but it happens often enough, and powerfully enough that leatherfolk seek it, at least subconsciously. Some, though, make it the "point" of their scene.

Scientists attribute such feelings to the release in our bodies of naturally-occurring chemicals called endorphins. Our bodies use them to block pain and, by their nature, they are pleasure-producing. I sense that there is more to this than meets the eye, or the microscope for that matter. What that may be eludes me, but fortunately the ecstacy hasn't.

The sensations of ecstacy may include feelings of flying, drifting, weightlessness, a sense that my body's "vibration" has risen substantially, or my senses being made more acutely aware of my surroundings. Not only do I sense surrounding "angels" but I know that I too share, in some way, that kind of existence as well.

Others talk of seeing vivid colors, hearing "heavenly" music, and experiencing soul travel. Several people have told me that they have left their bodies and hovered over the scene, watching the action from a distance, even as it was themselves they were watching!

3. Bonding

In an article published in "Newslink" (Spring 1993, Number 25), the quarterly newsletter of New York's Gay Male S/M Activists, Ron Gest writes about the value of that group's "Demo Nights":

"One of the great joys of s/m is the communication that can occur between two men, even in the confines of a demonstration. In some cases, the technique being demonstrated . . . is really the starting point for a complex interplay of sensuousness, emotion, and physicality far beyond my ability to put into words. But what I am capable of is seeing and sensing this happening between two men whose most basic needs are woven together in a sado-masochistic interplay of mutual satisfaction, pleasure-giving and fulfillment. When this happens a tremendous thing occurs. The participants need not be 'experts' with years of experience. As important as they are, technique and experience count for less than trust, emotional honesty, and 'giving' and 'letting go.'"

"I cannot imagine any better way to bond, to fulfill our own most deep felt needs, to joyously help fulfill the needs of someone we love. This is the essence of what our Activism is all about. . . Not many of our scenes look like they fell off the Sistine chapel (a few maybe) but, hey, when they occur, aren't these moments of intense closeness (oneness if you will) what we really want to get to?"

That's what we at least try to achieve. We're not always successful of course. There are many variables in the formula, and many reasons why a scene doesn't work. But take it from me, when it does, it's just as wonderful as we hoped, just as good as could be.

Chapter 8

WHY AM I DOING THAT TO HIM?

Bill asked me why I was a top. He wasn't being critical, just curious. After all, the whipping, tit play, and out-right domination doesn't seem very politically correct. My mom will tell you she didn't raise *me* that way.

My mastery goes against all that is sacred, accepted, and approved in contemporary Western culture. I wasn't taught to inflict pain, cause men to cry, and bruise (even lightly) bodies for my own gratification. On the other hand, some nuns did use rulers to good advantage; maybe I'm just following their example!

Seriously though, I have reasons for enjoying SM. Before I explain them, there is one overriding qualification I'd like to make clear: I am writing about safe, sane, and consensual behavior. There are no compromises in that regard.

Happily, a great deal of sadomasochistic activity falls into the category of safe and sane, so if you'll consent, I'll gladly do it.

Why? It gives me pleasure. I don't know why watching an ass turn red under a whip, or seeing a bottom grimace with pain turns me on, but it does. I find it exciting, erotic, and greatly stimulating. I like those feelings.

I like the feeling of control that my slaves give me. Whether simply to balance other aspects of my life, or because it's an expression of my personality, I enjoy control. Having a person obey me is pleasurable. When what he does for me is pleasurable and is done in obedience, the pleasure is intensified. As with much of the reasoning in this book, I can't readily explain it, but I can vouch for it as the way I feel.

At a discussion group I once attended, a dominatrix said she was a sadist because it made her bottoms feel good. That's not what we would expect a sadist to say, but there is a lot of truth in it.

We top because that's what bottoms want us to do. Being the dominant partner is being of service. Now I'll admit it's no kind of "Mother Theresa" labor, but it certainly is answering another's desires.

This is where the consensual part comes in. Whether the activity is agreed upon verbally or arrived at intuitively, it is gratifying to help your partner experience his or her fantasies. Opening the "door" to the bottom's wishes is both a privilege and a responsibility that carries its own reward.

I also enjoy the sense of discovery in the activity, learning as I watch what happens. For me, the wonder of seeing a bottom take it, or do it never ceases. I marvel at the strength of bottoms, their ability to submit, withstand, and create.

Additionally, there is vicarious experience being gained. I may not feel it in the same way as the bottom, but I enjoy it as I participate. It gratifies my voyeuristic self. I want to see the action unfold.

There's an exchange of energy in the play. Sometimes it is beneath (or beyond) our usual perceptions, but it is there nonetheless. At other times, the "electricity" or "magnetism" is undeniable. In any case, it influences and attracts us, bringing deep satisfaction, perhaps in ways about which we know nothing.

When we move beyond superficiality, we can develop a rare and beautiful intimacy. We become connected to each other, balancing each other as top and bottom, as pain and pleasure, yin and yang.

Next to the pleasure of sexual release, the shared space *afterwards* holds the most pleasure. When we are exhausted by the rough-housing, the sexual activity, the pain and the pleasure, we share moments of sublime quiet in each other's arms.

I have seen my partner in anguish and pain. I have pushed him to his very limits, challenging him to go beyond them, and he has. He has pleasured me as only a real submissive can. Both these aspects—mastery and submission—draw us together in a closeness seldom duplicated. Then, after the scene, or during a break in the action, we share feelings and sensations of deep peace. I can only hint at the "presence" surrounding such a time, but it's there.

There's more to leather activity than sex, but when sex is part of the scene, the sexual pleasure is increased by the intensity of the sadomasochism.

Chapter 9

DE SADE'S NOT INTO
THE LEATHER SCENE

Since I write a regular column about SM, I thought I'd do some historical research. I dutifully went out and purchased not one, but two books of writings by the Marquis de Sade: *The 120 Days of Sodom and Other Writings*, and *Justine, Philosophy in the Bedroom, and Other Writings*. Unless you're interested in the French Revolution, I don't recommend either volume.

Unfortunately, de Sade's characters give leather sadists a bad name. Of course, I guess they (OK, we) have a sorry reputation to begin with. After all, my dictionary defines sadism as "The perversion of deriving sexual satisfaction from the infliction of pain on others; Delight in cruelty." I remember that the sadists of my childhood were the guys who pulled wings off of butterflies.

I once paddled a friend's ass until it had a beautiful black and blue mark and pinched and clamped his tits until they were raw (but not bleeding) with pain. But I never pulled off butterfly wings.

I would like to coin a new name for leatherfolk such as myself, but I honestly can't think of one. One lesbian I know defined herself as a sadist. It went something like this: "I'm a sadist. I enjoy making others feel good."

What are the chances of storming the offices of Merriam Webster, and changing their definition to accommodate ours? Slim, I think.

The sadism of the leather community has little or nothing in common with the fantasies of the Marquis. Ours is both safe (his characters committed murder) and consensual (they kidnapped their underaged victims). If those distinctions aren't clear enough, we can add to them the fact that our "sadism" is for mutual pleasure. Rinella's dictionary would define sadism as "the use of pain-inducing actions in order to arouse another to a heightened state of pleasure."

A secondary effect of the activity is the pleasure the sadist receives as well.

There are both physical and psychological reasons why the masochist derives pleasure from the pain. Why the sadist derives pleasure is probably less evident. For myself, I find the infliction of pain on another (and at times on myself) sexually exciting. Paddling an ass, whipping a back, and clamping tits and genitals arouse me intensely. I am not alone. Once, I was at a local leather bar where just the *sound* of someone being paddled quickly attracted a large group of observers.

Of the over seventy columns I've written, none have gotten more responses than those about spanking. Pain is popular! Why that is the case is not easily deduced.

Misters Miriam and Webster would write it off as perversion, but I think otherwise. I think it has to do with wholeness.

Reasons such as curiosity, amazement, and stimulation are why we do such things. Fundamentally, though, sadism (and masochism) as defined in the leather community allow us to safely, sanely, and consensually explore our "Dark Sides." That is why I say "wholeness." To repress and deny that we have dark sides to our personalities is to deny stark and very "real" reality. To be Pollyanna is foolishness, dangerous foolishness at that.

Repressed, denied, hidden darkness only festers until it vents itself in some other way. Just as uncontrolled bliss, lightness, and goodness is unreasonable, un-experienced evil is an illusion. What we need is a balanced, healthy, and manageable dark event. Such experiences allow us to understand ourselves and our motivations, to give expression to those motives and, so, reduce their power and their drive.

My partner—in the scene mentioned at the beginning of this chapter—went home with a painful mark on his ass. The mark was only a sign of a more important inner event. He had come face to face with his own need for pain, had endured it, and—for reasons I'm not competent to explain—he had enjoyed it.

Every time I paused in the scene to check on his welfare (something the Marquis' characters never did) he was forceful in his expression of pleasure. When I took off the tit clamps whose unshielded metal teeth had bitten into his nipples, he writhed in pain, only to say how "great" it felt.

I don't understand it. I'm not talking about a fool or a jerk. My friend is a systems analyst with a successful career in a major computer firm. He is educated, mature, financially stable. He is new to the SM scene but finds that it has eliminated the boredom previously present in his sex life. He likes what happens with a leather master.

And what is it my friend responds to? It is pleasure. As Race Bannon writes in his book, *Learning the Ropes* (Dacdalus Publishing Company, 1992), "When the S/M community adopted the safe, sane and consensual credo, I was overjoyed. It serves its purpose well. But I've always thought it lacked one thing—fun.

"S/M is supposed to be fun. If it weren't, why would anyone do it? So I want to add the word 'fun' to the credo . . . By doing so, you'll insure yourself not only safe experiences, but fun and fulfilling ones as well."

Sadists in the leather community then are those who inflict pleasure. It is pleasure of an intense degree, skillfully induced with necessary caution, measured speed, and careful recognition of the masochist's responses.

To remain faithful to the credo of safe, sane, and consensual, the sadist cannot be unaware of the bottom, or be self-centered in his or her pursuit of pleasure. In fact, the center of the sadist's attention must be the recipient of the sadistic activity.

"How is this affecting my partner?" is the sadist's ultimate and continuous concern. Pausing for feedback, listening for breathing patterns, feeling for numbness or coolness in the extremities, and being aware of possible abrasions and cuts in the skin are all ways that a leather sadist protects the bottom.

I knew what effect those metal teeth were having—after all, they've bitten my tits at times as well—and I knew that my partner found them pleasurable. He had told me so, and if the situation had not been enjoyable it would have ended.

The leather sadist uses learned skills and appropriate technique. Pain is administered slowly, its intensity built. Explicitly pleasurable activity, such as kissing and caressing, is interspersed with more direct pain. Rest periods allow the bottom to adjust to increased levels of intensity. The sadist continuously encourages the bottom, offering advice, instructions, and support in the bottom's effort to transmute the pain into pleasure. The sadist reinforces the positive and builds the bottom's self-esteem. In short, the leather sadist cares.

Until we find a better word, we're stuck with the name sadist, but other than that we have very little in common with the old Marquis' fiction. That's too bad for his characters. They missed a grand amount of pleasure, and that's the point of sadism in the first place. So, have a great time, but please don't pull off any butterfly's wings!

Chapter 10

IDEAS FOR A MASTERS' MANUAL

Attitude makes the difference between being a master and a top. Technique, desire, experience, and a bottom's willingness to serve contribute to a master's role, of course. But in the long run, what distinguishes a real master from those folks who are playing at it is attitude. Just as the right attitude is crucial for being "best boy," a master's mindset creates his ability to take, exercise, and keep control. Service and pleasure are certainly a master's reward, but the number one desire of a master must be to be in control.

Masters don't grab and wrestle for control either. Instead they see their partners' submission as a freely given gift, and their domination of another as simply fulfilling the others' needs. Despite the fact that many young men and women try to dominate (and in many ways succeed), it really takes practice to be able to command another. I still believe that only the best bottoms make it to the top. "Going bottom" provides insight into the meaning of service, the effect of pain, and the altered states that submission allows a slave to enter.

Someday I'd like to marshal the resources necessary for establishing an academy for masters and slaves. Until then, here are "Rinella's Six Attributes Every Master Needs."

1. Self-Confidence.

What a person thinks of himself contributes to the image others have of him. It's a matter, then, of knowing that you are a master/mistress. Self doubt, poor self esteem, and anxiety translate into unclear signals, hesitation, and confusion.

Gaining self-confidence is no easy matter. It takes self-examination and a clear appraisal of oneself. Generally it is a gift of time, since positive, affirming experiences as a top build the confidence needed to be the master that you want to be.

2. Trustworthiness.

The frequency with which the word trust appears in leatherfolks' conversations is no accident. It is the basis of successful relationships—of leather relationships no less than any others. Be trustworthy and your submissive(s) will obey and serve. Deceit and cunning will insure that you will receive the same in return.

Prior to starting any scene, and certainly as the scene continues, (hopefully) growing into a relationship, build trust and prove you are trustworthy. I often tell those who submit to me, "The more you trust me, the more I can get away with." And it is true. There isn't a single SM activity that doesn't depend upon and benefit from mutual trust.

3. Consistency.

How the master acts sets the example and teaches the slave how to be. Masters who change their minds, live double standards, and say one thing while doing another can't take control. For a slave to submit, there has to be a framework in which he/she can "know the rules" and develop dependable expectations. Arbitrary and ambivalent actions indicate a lack of self-confidence.

4. Responsibility.

As a master whom I respect a great deal once said, "It's

the slave's responsibility to serve. The master is responsible for the relationship." Be decisive. Know what you want and make your wishes known. Likewise, be responsible for your actions and for your slave(s). That means take care.

Taking care is more than being careful, though. It means to protect your slave and watch for his/her physical safety. Domination, sadism, and the inflicting of pain are the master's prerogative. Keeping the slave free from injury and harm are the master's duty.

5. Acceptance.

Mastery and the world of leathersex are unacceptable lifestyles in modern America. But unless a master accepts his position, he will forever be merely playing a role. Real mastery of others depends upon one's ability to accept the service, the attention, and the submission that a slave wants, needs, and desires to give.

To be comfortable with the idea of domination and/or sadism, one must see oneself as worthy of such attention. Doing that, of course, means that you can see your mastery within the context of a wider world view. The master I quoted before, for instance, believes that all life is a circle. It is a personal philosophy that allows him to see all "sides" of life on the same plane. It is a viewpoint more Eastern than most, as we Westerners see duality where others (such as Buddhists) see the inherent unity in opposites (yin and yang).

However you synthesize your thoughts and feelings about SM, until you accept yourself as who you are, there will be a struggle that will make true realization of your Self difficult, if not impossible.

6. Expertise.

Experience is the best teacher and good technique is

53

crucial to success. I can't give you either of them in these pages, but there are ways to learn and grow. Avail yourself of any of the several groups that teach good SM practices. Find a master you can learn from and make yourself his willing student. Read, discuss, ask questions, get answers.

It's a challenge to be a good master. The benefits are both exciting and satisfying. And the leather scene needs good masters. I encourage you to go for all you aspire to be. Make the investment in yourself to reach your fantasies. Your slave will thank you.

Chapter 11

A NATURAL SENSE
OF BALANCE

Scientists say that all things tend towards equilibrium, which the dictionary defines as "a condition in which all acting influences are canceled by others, resulting in a stable, balanced, or unchanging system." It's not so much that that state is attained, but, like a swinging pendulum, balance is kept. As soon as an object veers too far one way, it returns to the middle, if only on its way to the other extreme.

Over the years, I have been amazed at the non-sexual, non-leather aspects of those into sado-masochism. Contrary to popular wisdom, the leather world is inhabited by those we'd least expect to indulge in such fantasies. Doctors, lawyers, ministers, judges, successful and powerful men and women from all walks of life share SM experiences.

I don't have the statistical data necessary to prove my point, but having met hundreds of leather tops and bottoms, I am sure that their average education is higher, their incomes greater, and their power and authority well above that of the statistical American norm.

Why does a prosperous, intelligent, and successful person enter the "dark" world of leathersex? To regain and maintain his balance. Let me cite a favorite example:

Charles is a loan officer at a major metropolitan bank. He is responsible for the management of loan portfolios worth millions of dollars. He grants or denies credit to fortune 500 corporations throughout the Midwest. He is wined and dined by men of power and prestige. Yet, when he enters his leather world, it is as a collared dog-slave. He eats from a bowl on the floor and gives his master whatever pleasure his master requires.

His two lives are in complete juxtaposition. Each of them is real, vibrant, and fulfilling. Each balances the other and makes the other possible, desirable, and sustainable. Some call it escapism, but it can be a viable alternative to stress, pressure, and self-destruction. Show me a one-sided coin. None exists. The round Yin-Yang symbol, with its equal and contrasting white/black design illustrates the principle of complimentary balance.

When the master or mistress reddens an ass with whips and paddles, he or she is dominant, aggressive, and assertive of power, realizes the warrior side of the self. And if this aspect of self is down-trodden, ignored, or denied in other areas of life—at work or in family, for example—in a leather scene it can be exercised and allowed to grow. Likewise, when a controlling, directing, and powerful individual relinquishes those aspects of self by becoming, for whatever short span of time, an obedient, submissive, and worshipping servant, he or she regains balance. In either case the end result is often a catharsis of delightful proportions.

Because of the self-defined and mutually accepted limits of leathersex (i.e., safe, sane, and consensual), emotions, fears, anxieties, and pressures may be released in a structured, supportive, practical, and non-destructive way. What makes this balancing activity more interesting is to observe it over the course of time. The real phenomenon is that one's leathersex activities change as other elements in one's environment vary.

In my own life, when my career shifted into areas of less authority, less pay, and less responsibility, my sex life became more dominant. Later, as I found my needs to dominate satisfied and as my income increased and my personal power improved, I began looking for someone to serve.

In writing, it appears (I hope) that all of this is very well-thought out. In truth, our actions can be as mystifying as the universe. Reflection and dialogue may reveal some of our motives, may explain part of what's going on, but we only understand in part. Simply put, I don't have all the answers—and your usual leathersex scene is much more physical, more emotional, and more earthy than will ever be recounted in print. After all, in spite of anyone's pontification, the first goal is pleasure. We do this because it's fun.

Over time and with experience, you'll find added dimensions in dungeon play. The balance that we naturally seek brings us into wholeness. The most satisfying scenes recognize, each in its own way, the uniqueness of the participants and the various ways they experience themselves and each other physically, mentally, emotionally, and spiritually.

There is love and lust, pain and pleasure, sensory overload and sensory deprivation. In the end, the best scenes bring balance, a strange and quiet state of inner rest. It may sound corny to say it, but when all is done, there remains a peace that hums within, even as we re-enter our lives and the pendulum swings on.

57

Chapter 12

LEATHER LIT. 101

Nobody's surprised when I say that there weren't a whole lot of leatherfolk in the small Indiana city where I came out as a leatherman. I got a lot of my early SM experiences because I traveled for a living. In my home town there were two guys who showed me the ropes and taught me about the business end of a paddle. But there was a lot more to my "education" than raw sex. Fact is, much of it came from books and magazines.

My first leather-style relationship used *Mr. Benson*, (Bad Boy Press, New York, 1992), a novel by John Preston, as a guide. My slave at the time was expected to live and care for me as Jamie would for Mr. Benson.

Like everyone else, I had read Larry Townsend's *Leatherman's Handbook* (current edition: LT Publications, Los Angeles, CA, 1993). Truth is, I'm old enough to have read the first (1972) edition. Its scenes turned me on. Its instructions are as valid today as they were then. Years later, the things I was only reading about have been proven true by experience.

George Stambolian's *Male Fantasies/Gay Realities*, (The Sea Horse Press, New York, 1984) wasn't exactly a book about leather, but his chapter interviewing the masochist gave me a perspective on dominance and submission that helped overcome my fears of being a top. The book is good for anyone coming out, and it has occasional passages that refer to leather.

One of the most important books in Leather Lit is *Urban Aboriginals*, by Geoff Mains, (Gay Sunshine Press, San Francisco, 1984). Geoff originally wrote this as a master's thesis, but don't let that stop you from reading it. He's done a thorough (if now a bit dated) research into gay SM. His understandings and explanations include physiology, psychology, sociology, and a lot of really hot men.

You won't pass leather Lit 101 without reading *Urban Aboriginals*.

I write about *The Exchange* by Robert Payne in chapter 19 so I won't comment on it here, but I do recommend it.

When it comes to authors I've read and re-read, John Preston tops the list. His work is erotic, informative, and instructional. His fiction holds one's attention, causes positive, groin-centered reactions, and gives the mind explanations, insights, and ideas all at the same time.

I've already mentioned John Preston's classic, *Mr. Benson*. The same author's *I Once Had a Master* (Alyson Publications, Boston, 1984) is another of those books that originally turned me on to leather. It is primarily a novice's journey into leather. This series of short stories is a good chance to see how one character becomes progressively more accustomed to seeing himself as a leatherman. His fictional journey is not uncommon in leather life.

For the Love of a Master (Alyson, Boston, 1987) and *In Search of a Master* (Alyson, Boston, 1988)—also from Preston's "Master" series—make wonderful reading as well. Not only are they great stroke books but they have plot, character, humor, and insight. They present the world of the "Network." Here the wealthy buy and sell men and women who have freely indentured themselves as sexual submissives. Those who would sell their sexual service are trained and groomed to please the most demanding request. It is all properly covered by contracts, rights are protected, intimate pleasures sold. Slavery in America? I can't help but believe that it happens. I'd like to get an invitation to the Auction (and, of course, to have the necessary funds to do some bidding).

Entertainment for a Master, also by Preston, (Alyson, Boston, 1986) is the story of a party the narrator held in San Francisco. It reads as if it could be true, and if it isn't, it should have been.

A bit more esoteric (but far less fictional) is Jack Morin's *Anal Pleasure & Health*. Anal eroticism is hardly limited to the leather scene. This book, written by a Ph.D. gives lots of ideas and practical suggestions, especially about fucking and fisting. It answers questions that most of us are too shy to ask.

In the area of purely delicious erotica and a bit further from mainstream leather is the Beauty trilogy by Anne Rice writing as A. N. Roquelaure. *The Claiming of Sleeping Beauty*, *Beauty's Punishment*, and *Beauty's Release* (Penguin Books, New York, 1983) will keep all of you warm this winter, no matter how cold the winds blow. Like Preston's fiction, the Beauty trilogy offers sensuality with insight. It is pure fantasy set in some ancient European Kingdom where the aristocracy surrenders its young adult princes and princesses to sexual slavery. These books offer a fictional, but enlightening, viewpoint on pain and pleasure, submission and desire.

Mineshaft Nights by Leo Cardini (First Hand Books, Teaneck, NJ, 1990) is a series of short stories about what may have been leather's hottest bar. It's set in the days when sleazy sex was still safe, and there is plenty of sleaze to go around. It's fiction, but there's more truth in it than most Sunday-school teachers will ever believe.

Another book by Larry Townsend, *Masters' Counterpoint* (Alyson, Boston, 1991) proves that good SM can also have a good story line. This mystery novel, complete with sex, psychology, and realistic narrative, has enough SM to make my list, but will be appreciated by mainstream readers as well.

Ties That Bind (Daedalus Publishing Company, Los Angeles, 1993) by International Mr. Leather 1989, Guy Baldwin, is a compilation of the author's insightful, and sometimes controversial columns from *Drummer* and other leather magazines. In this book, Baldwin takes a deep and genuine look at the modern leather world. His observations contain a great deal of reason and sanity, especially in the area of SM relationships. This book is essential reading if you want to get deeply involved in a master/slave coupling.

Race Bannon's *Learning the Ropes* (Daedalus Publishing Company, Los Angeles, 1992), is, as the cover says, "A Basic Guide To Safe And Fun S/M Lovemaking."

Other books that should be mentioned, but don't rate as high on my list are *Leather Blues* by Jack Fritscher (Gay Sunshine Press), *The Corporal in Charge of Taking Care of Captain O'Malley* (Gay Sunshine Press, 1984), *Leathermen Speak Out*, edited by Jack Ricardo (Leyland Publications, San Francisco, 1991), and *The Brig* (not for the faint hearted—and out of print anyway).

It may be near the end of my list, but *Leatherfolk*, edited by Mark Thompson (Alyson Publications, Boston, 1992), is very near to my heart. As a reviewer in *Manifest Reader* wrote "It's sexy, startling, informative and challenging. It starts where we live—in our leathers—and takes off on an explanation of the realms where sex magic meets spirituality."

Most of these books can be ordered by mail from the publishers or through your favorite bookstore.

Chapter 13

SOMETIMES MASTER, SOMETIMES SLAVE

The leather community makes a big deal out of the roles one chooses to play. Top, bottom, and versatile are tags we apply to each other and ourselves with an easy frequency. Less often, but just as categorically, we choose the titles of master or slave.

When I write my "Leather Views" column, I write as a leatherman who generally 'goes top' but always keeps an eye open to meet that *perfect* master who will lead me to ecstacy—or, at least, give me one hell of a good time. But, as most bottoms will be quick to point out, good tops are hard to find, so most of my experiences are on the side of domination.

Humans, of course, don't fit into the clean molds of leather stereotypes. The truth is that in some way or another, each of us, including the most dominant master and the most experienced slave, is versatile. Versatility is simply the recognition of potential.

Early in my leather career, while feeling very much that I was a top, I vacationed in the Rocky Mountains. There I met a ruggedly handsome, strong, and vibrant man. We spent an evening in front of his fireplace. I fell in love (unfortunately a fleeting event) and in that moment felt I could be his slave forever. So much for being a top! Leather roles are determined not by code but by relationship.

A young man once left me a message, and when I called him back we began to talk about roles. He was new to the scene, and pointed out that he wanted to learn how to be a bottom. He quickly emphasized that his desire only applied to his sex life, since in every other area he wanted to and did remain in control.

His comment demonstrated how we over-simplify the ways we relate. We want to closely define types and make everything "black or white." If we can label it, we can understand it. But the world doesn't work that way. Just when we think we have the answers, there are new questions. There are neither tops, nor bottoms, just men and women who choose to enter into relationships that, to some degree or another, fulfill their need for dominance or submission, being served or serving.

Our cultural baggage assigns value to various roles, powerful ones being "better" and subservient ones being "worse." By the structure of our society, to be top is desirable and slavery denotes failure.

Is my writing more credible since I "come off" as a top? What if Jack Rinella were someone's slave? What kind of value judgement do you place on that? Can a hot looking woman be submissive? Can a fat ugly man be a master? Is there really a better or lesser role?

Experiential truth contradicts common wisdom. A good top is careful, reading body language, sensing how his bottom is reacting. He takes care not to do damage. His goal is mutual pleasure—and if that is arrived at through the application of pain, then it is careful, appropriate, and desired, not forced, damaging, or in anger. In a word, it works!

Very often, it is the bottom who is in control and

directing the scene.

And these roles are not fixed, they change as we mature. They change as we meet new people. Likewise, our sexual modality may be quite different from what we are in other arenas.

A person who dominates us sexually, may have an egalitarian relationship with us in other areas of our life. Masters and slaves often take on those roles only at home, or—even in private—they may restrict the roles to specific time periods or certain rooms. The slave in the bedroom might be the one in charge of the checkbook or the one who plans vacations and social engagements.

It would be a lot easier if it were all "cut and dried," but it isn't. No matter how much fantasy is involved, no matter how much we want it to be one way or the other, our relationships are dynamic and interactive.

The young man who wanted to find a top questioned how he could find someone he could trust to tie him up. There is no short answer. The interpersonal skills necessary in school or family or work are the same skills needed between top and bottom.

The differences we see in the leather world are only differences of degree. Yes, there is more intensity. Yes, it is a radical lifestyle, out of the accepted norm. But that doesn't change the fact that the participants are human, warm, thinking, feeling, acting, and reacting.

Why a person goes one way or the other is anyone's guess. How they relate to you is up to you since we are talking about people, real people with real feelings. We are talking about relationships, some of long duration, others short lived perhaps, but no less real.

When we no longer look upon each other as objects, as actors who play assigned roles, we will be closer to meaningful and satisfactory relationships in all areas of living—and that includes leather.

Chapter 14

THE QUESTION OF EQUALITY

Aristotle wrote that some men were born "natural slaves;" our Founding Fathers wrote that "All men are created equal." While some men and women may revel in the sight of a collared slave licking a master's boot, others shy away from the idea.

A hot-looking Daddy type once told me of a night at a local leather bar. He was standing at the bar when he saw a master whisper something to his slave-companion, and hand him his leash. Seconds later the slave was at my friend's side asking to lick his boots. "I know it would have been a turn-on for both master and slave. I know I should have let him do it, but it just wasn't anything I could let happen. I had to send the disappointed boy back with a 'Thanks, but no thanks.'" This just proves the obvious: Not everyone in a leather bar is into the same kind of scene.

Usually though, dominance and submission are integral to what happens in leathersex. In spite of appearances to the contrary, I'd like to make the point that domination doesn't necessarily obliterate equality. The leather community is egalitarian in as much as it is often and generally ruled by respect. We who linger on the outer limits and those who venture beyond, have a code of respect for each other. I dare say that it is the "rugged individualist" of SM that understands best that equality is more than simply being equal, that mutual respect is not a desire for sameness, and that independence leaves no room for identical identities.

The problem posed in the equality discussion is that it is difficult to admit to differences without implying degrees of quality. We easily perceive a master as "better" than a slave—but at what price? What cultural baggage demands that higher rank is better rank? Why do we assume that less power (when accepted willingly, embraced happily) is inferior to greater power?

When confronted with the idea of submission as a lower state, I think of the men I have known who have served. They have been strong, courageous men. Any Saturday night in a leather bar proves my point. In spite of living in a culture based on dominance, power, and coercion, more than half the men at any given leather function are pleased to submit. In fact they're disappointed if they can't. The preponderance of wanna-be slaves attests to the real nature of submission. It sets on end the notion of equality.

When I first met a man I could serve, there was no thought of who's better, or should we (could we) be equal? Instead, I was filled with an overwhelming sense of awe at his power and poise. I desired to worship him. He stirred in me feelings of fulfillment and completion that made some deep, hidden font spring to life. As it turned out, the encounter was all too short-lived, but I will never forget how fine it felt to be slavish. What most discussions on SM and equality omit is the more important idea of fulfillment and satisfaction.

The modern day notion of equality demands some kind of conformity to a standard, to some approved bench-mark of what is better. But in fact, many qualities are neither better nor worse. Is it better to be short or tall? Dark or fair? There is no ranking of real power or real service. Of itself power is neutral. The roles we play or the roles we live are neither better nor worse. Their goodness, their rightness springs from the intention, the purpose of our hearts. The real bench-mark is the standard of our souls.

When my friend declined the offered boot-licking he was being neither better nor worse. He was being true to his own feelings. That strong Daddy, grey-haired, slightly heavy, sincerely smiling, is every bit as much a leatherman as the master/slave pair that invited him into their fantasy. And that fantasy spoke nothing of the reality of their after-the-bars relationship, the equality in their life together the next day. Who could tell which of them paid the bills, who made the decisions, or how they related in non-leather areas of their lives? And they, on their part, were being true to the drum beat they heard. For master and slave are not degrees on the scale of goodness. They are the same degree. They are both good in so far as they reflect the inner goodness and just desires of the doer.

The leather community may (in its best aspects) be the most egalitarian of all sub-cultures, for it allows us, as far as we dare, to the explore the inner selves we dream to be.

We certainly have the capacity to be more or less, better or worse. Though we often compare each to the other, in reality the only comparison that matters is how we measure up to our own potential. Do I want to be equal? You bet I do. I want to be equal to the best me that I am. When each of us is equal to our best selves, there'll be no need for any other kind of equality. The question will have been forever answered.

71

Chapter 15

MAKING IT MORE
THAN INTERESTING

Frank said his first leather scene was "interesting," a word I use every once in a while. The American Heritage Dictionary defines it as "arousing or holding attention; absorbing." I often use the word in situations that make me think, or satisfy my curiosity. But, I associate other feelings with interesting as well, and I suspect that Frank's answer veiled deeper feelings of disappointment. Even when I'm interested, I can feel moments of fear or boredom.

Frank brought a well-defined set of expectations to his first leather scene (it was bondage). Years of fantasy had given him time to imagine an event that he looked to the top to create for him. The top, for his part, could only do so much, given the fact that he and Frank were strangers. It's hard enough to get inside a person's head when you know him. With a first-time partner, it's nearly impossible.

So Frank got tied up. Honestly, the scene wasn't bad. There was no pain, little discomfort, and it was interesting. But we use different bench-marks. We look for excitement and orgasmic fire-works. We expect our partner to give us an experience that launches us into orbit forever. It's the other's job to give us bliss that never ends.

And therein lies the fallacy.

Oh, yes, there is bliss. Ecstacy can be had. But there is

a price to pay and that price is abandonment.

The coffee mug cartoon says it plainly enough: "Love is letting go of fear." What we need to abandon is our expectations, our fear, our self-doubt. We need to let go of our plans and release ourselves from the hold that determines "this is what will happen." When we do that—and it is not easily done—we can discover the world without boundaries wherein lies bliss.

The essential ingredient, of course, is trust. In discussing his first time, Frank admitted to one moment where freedom broke through. He was tied to a chair, naked, aroused, arms secured behind him, his legs roped apart. The top shoved his hairy chest into Frank's face. Frank began to gently suck on the guy's nipple. He turned his attention to that "lucky tit" and, as he did so, Frank began to drift. It was a taste of what he wanted. It was more than interesting. But it didn't last long, perhaps only long enough to show Frank he was going in the right direction, his efforts *could* be rewarded. He could trust having a nipple to suck on. It was familiar territory. The ropes and chains weren't. Neither was the room nor the top.

Let's explore the issue of trust further, as Frank and I did in our conversation. It is obvious that there can be no scene without trust. He had waited years to find someone he could trust. Fear-filled images of pain, disease, humiliation at the hand of some leather-clad sex-maniac were constantly thwarting his search for an opportunity to be tied up.

He wanted to know how you could trust someone. "You need first to trust yourself," I answered. We are the prime creators of our experiences. It's not fear of others, but fear of ourselves that hinders bliss. Self-doubt is often in control. We have the information we need to evaluate any situation. The universe is full of clues: advice from friends, our gut reaction, the other's verbal responses and body language, intuition, common sense.

When the Dahmer tragedy hit the newspapers, my friend Lee asked me if I wasn't at risk by going to leather bars. "Wouldn't you have gone home with Dahmer?" he asked. Simple fact is that I wouldn't because common sense tells me not to go home with someone whose drinking is out of control.

Society puts a heavy (but not unmanageable) trip on us that often causes us to suffer from poor self-images. As we accept their cultural put-downs, we accept the limitations that they place on us and so see ourselves as untrustworthy. But we can learn to trust ourselves and, when we do, we don't have to worry about trusting anyone else. When we trust ourselves, we listen to ourselves and know what to do. That information may be to do nothing, may be to avoid that situation, or to embrace it for everything it's worth.

When we can release ourselves from self-doubt, we can accept the universe for the blessing it is. When we trust ourselves we know we can handle anything life sends our way. And *that* brings me back to abandonment. Each of the great religions speak of the need to lose one's life in order to save it. It is the paradox of this planet that holding tight to something strangles it, setting it free lets it return to us more closely.

When I am master, I do so fully, totally. I allow myself to enter completely into the mindset. When I go bottom, I do the same. I trust myself to know what to do. I listen to myself and do what I think/feel/know is best. When in doubt, I do without. When Frank learns to do the same, all of his life, not just his sexual encounters, will be more than "interesting."

Chapter 16

IT'S A MATTER OF TRUST

Chuck and I spent three hours one day talking about his problems. Seems he can't make up his mind about SM. It's a long time fantasy that he has never fulfilled. He just can't decide what to do. Fact is, he can't make up his mind in many areas of his life. Should he move to a better neighborhood? Go back to school? Find a better job? And if he finds an answer, how will he know it's the right answer?

So I began talking about trusting oneself, just as I wrote in the last chapter. But that chapter about trust is too theoretical. Yes it is true, but it doesn't give any guidelines as to *how* to learn to trust yourself. Let me try to make up that deficiency.

Isn't it a matter of trusting others, not yourself?

Not entirely. Trusting another depends on trusting one's own perceptions and conclusions. Confusion sets in not because we don't trust others, but because we don't trust our own ability to decide whom to trust and whom not to trust. So to find someone to trust, we've first got to have faith in our being able to do so.

And that's why the trust that matters is in oneself.

Though I risk sounding more like a New Age guru than a leatherman, the first suggestion I have is to meditate on a regular basis. Choose your own style: lake-side walks or classical music, mantras, easy chairs, professionally produced tapes, or total silence. The *how* of regular reflection is not nearly as important as the activity itself.

Everyday, our brain passes through multiple levels of activity. Some peaceful, most hectic and scrambled. Our routine waking state is fairly busy as thoughts and feelings dart about in our mind. In times of deep relaxation we move into *alpha states*. It is at this alpha level that we begin to get in touch with our trustworthy inner self. There are plenty of books that explain various methods of meditation. Personally, I use a mixture of practices, some of which are my own discoveries—but they work for me and that is what is important. I encourage you to find what works for you.

Both extroverts (who think by listening to themselves talk) and introverts (who talk after they've thought) have a need for counsel. A friend, therapist, minister, or lover presents an opportunity for reflective interaction. Find someone who will be non-directive, supportive, and challenging in a non-critical way. The best thing he or she can do is ask you the questions you ought to be asking yourself.

The next step is research. Ask questions, read books, watch videos, go someplace where the information is and find it. The process mustn't stop at just an intellectual research project. Real conclusions come from exploration. And here is the first step with real risk. Of course, find ways to reduce the risk, but unless one looks, one will never find. Experiment a little bit.

Chuck was stuck in the rut of needing complete assurance. He wanted to know in some absolute way what was the *best* course of action. Lacking that, he did nothing and remained stuck.

I'm not saying to go "whole hog," but there are

acceptable trade offs. Every action has an acceptable level of risk. People drown in bath tubs but thankfully that doesn't stop the rest of us from bathing. Too often we over-estimate the risk and its potential danger. We err on the side of inactivity, slowing down the process of growth and positive change.

You can't alter a sailboat's course unless it is moving. You can turn the wheel of a car all you want, but if it's parked it will still point in its original direction.

Experimentation, then, gives us experience. Having sampled the small deed, we are in a better situation to evaluate. If it didn't meet our expectations we can use the experience to settle the question. Once and for all, we will know that it's not for us. There'll be no more rumination and regret—the matter will be settled.

On the other hand, it just may be what we really wanted. Having taken the first step we now have more information, and are better able to continue our decision-making process. At this point we find ourselves back at reflection—another name for meditation—and the process continues. New answers most often lead to new questions. New questions to new searches. New searches to new discoveries and new questions.

In their own ways, the whips and chains and the paddles and clamps, the leather and the lifestyle have led me to all sorts of self discoveries and their own kinds of enlightenment.

Most importantly though, the lesson I've learned that has spoken the loudest is the that I can learn to trust myself. I can find my limits and my desires, and travel paths unique and fulfilling to me. If leather is the beat of a different drum then it is my drum that I hear, uniquely in tune for me. Listen to your own drum beat. It is a rhythm

79

that will free your soul.

Chapter 17

THE THIN LAYER
OF CIVILIZATION

Twentieth Century Americans consider themselves cultured, civilized, and far removed from the passions and animal urges of primitive mankind. But scratch the skin of any one of us, and you'll find a primal beast. Scratch it the wrong way, and you have the riots of Los Angeles. Let it rip at its worst, and you have the ovens of Nazi Germany. The fact remains that our thin layer will be scratched. For all our centuries of culture, we are still clad in a civilization that is merely a thin veneer.

I believe that the heart of mankind is beautiful. Goodness and kindness flow in our veins. Yet realism, my years of reading the daily newspaper, of walking past the panhandlers, of hearing crying children, all reveal a human condition not as pleasant as we might wish.

New Age gurus speak of mankind's dark side; Catholics call it original sin. Name it what you will, deny it if you like, but lurking beneath the veneer is danger. We live in a world that represses that danger, allowing it to simmer and rage in quiet desperation.

We are not allowed to feel. It is wrong to be angry. There is no space for the revelations of base instinct in today's sanitized world. But they remain there nevertheless, and they will confront us more often than we want.

Therein lies the advantage of leather.

Leather, in each of its various scenes, lets us get in touch with the primal issues of life and death, fear and bravery, violence and peace. It hearkens to a primitive, basic, corporal existence—almost (but not quite) the law of the jungle. The attraction, unspoken perhaps, that leather holds is both its contradiction to societal norms and the primal impulses it satisfies.

Naked bodies in heat. Pain and pleasure. Brute force and sweat. Leather and chains. The struggle of bondage, the reddened ass in a whipping scene, the service of a slave to his mistress. Each of these brings us into contact with deep and often hidden desires. They are passions too intense for a polite, law-abiding democracy, but they are real. To deny them is to deny our inner selves, to say we have no dark side. To express them wantonly is to court disaster.

Society has pushed these primal urges to hunt, conquer, dominate, to flee, surrender, serve, far from its respectable pretenses. Yet they lie not far below the board room table or the cafeteria lunch counter. Denied expression, they rear their ugly heads in spousal beating, child abuse, addictions, power plays and other forms of "acceptable" violence. Leather offers their release without the destruction they might otherwise cause.

As one of my readers once said, "I like leather because it is permissive. People into leather live and let others live as well. They may not like my fetish, but they respect me enough to let me practice it without criticism."

In fact, leather offers more than a permissive space. It supports and gives a framework in which to explore one's feelings, one's fantasies. The three guidelines of safe, sane, and consensual, maintain safety yet create a broad platform on which to experience the dark side of life. In leather, fantasies can happen, new realities can be explored. The animal rages and faces its prey. The Warrior fights and is fought. The Victor overcomes—or meets defeat in the process. Fears are faced and thereby vanquished. Experiencing one's limits, anguish, alternate ego, and suppressed desires is a learning and cleansing process. We face our fear, our selves, our lusts and our power. Our deeply hidden drives find expression. So we resolve our doubts and passions, giving vent to them and bringing them into a manageable, understandable light.

The dungeon is no place for therapy, the whipping post no place to work out one's anger, but there are deep feelings that do find safe, protected, controlled expression. We release our fears, our passions, when we don our leathers.

Many a bottom has smiled on Monday morning as he or she sat at an office desk, the pain on their asses still lingering. They know what most of their co-workers may never learn: we can live our fantasies and face our fears. The real self can emerge from behind the mask of culture. As fully functioning members of American society, we can find the equilibrium between beauty and the beast. Our primal selves can be as much a part of reality as the facade of day-to-day living. I may put aside my harness to go to school, or I may shed my dog collar before I get on the train on Monday morning, but the inner me still prospers as I find my limits, my self, and the true depth of my power.

Chapter 18

POWER

The introduction to this book lists the two "qualities that make a leatherman: proper technique and the right attitude." It goes on to say: "Being a master is not just one thing . . . but a mindset."

Fundamentally, those who aspire to be masters and mistresses must be comfortable with power. That means they need the ability to acquire it, use it, live with its consequences, to overcome the negative connotations inherent in being powerful, and to elude the corruption it may bring and the conceit it is liable to engender.

To do so can be difficult. The Judaeo-Christian ethic that permeates our culture inculcates us with a great deal of negativity about power. We are taught that the meek shall inherit the earth, that modesty and humility are virtues, and to turn the other cheek.

At the same time, our education fills us with ambivalence, for it reinforces in us the drive to compete, to win, to conquer, to gain fame and fortune by succeeding, while trying to insure that we are good, "law-abiding" citizens, i.e., that we do what we are told. It is kept a secret that success may be built on the backs of others who have failed.

As I reflect on the contents of this book, I smile to think of what I have become. In terms of career, the most significant teacher I ever had was an elderly nun. I learned writing skills from a liberal "brother" who at the time was frocked in black, wore a Roman collar, and attended Catholic Mass daily. Henry F., listed with them in the acknowledgements, was no less a dedicated Christian, loyal to his church, committed to the Gospel.

Such faith and commitment have their place and their own kind of power. In my mind, they pose no contradictions. I can't say the same for the common religionist's view of leather. If you are to succeed as a master, you too must resolve the conflicts and find your truth. That is the ultimate challenge.

We have been socialized from birth to eschew power. Society, of course, is ambivalent in that requirement: we honor the powerful wealthy, we elect politicians to power, we obey the power of our religious leaders. At the same time, most people accept their own powerlessness.

I, on the contrary, exhort you to claim your right to dominate, to rule, in fact, to enslave. (If only Abraham Lincoln could see me now!) To do that, you must first claim yourself. If you can not rule yourself, you can not rule others. A master needs to be comfortable with what it means to control another. Masters are responsible, directive, decisive. They need to be able to accept service, attention, the "gift of self" that a slave desires to bestow on his or her owner.

I once interviewed a master about his thoughts and feelings about having a slave. Not surprisingly, the man who considered himself a master, spoke assuredly, with a steady voice. He was relaxed in the interview and structured in his view of leather.

Listen to what he had to say:

What does it mean to be a master?

To accept responsibility for the relationship. A master,

other than just being dominant, is a balance for his slave who isn't just a bottom, but is one who really desires to serve. It's always seemed important to me that there be a balance, that the slave desired to serve as much as the master desired to command.

In practical terms what does being a master entail?

Understanding that you have control, which I think is difficult for most people. I think it's something that you have to experience.

It's the same kind of feeling you get now when you go someplace and there's a butler. Even though the person is a paid professional, it's difficult for most of us to understand what that relationship is, and what it means, and why a person would be happy as a butler.

You need to experience it to understand it.

Do you have a slave now? And what does that mean to you?

Yes, I do, and it means that I've found someone with whom to share that experience. Someone who understands the "flip side" of what I understand a master/slave relationship to be. It means someone has given himself as a gift whom I've accepted to use for my pleasure. Someone to learn and grow with, to share that whole master/slave relationship.

Where do you think that your mastery is going? What do you envision you're going to learn? What do you want to learn?

So much of the master/slave relationship is understanding the use of control. That's not something that comes easily for people.

Professionally, I do a lot of activities where I control large numbers of people. But doing that in a sexual way over one or two special people entails a different mindset altogether. They spring from the same root but they are different portions of the same activity.

Does that mean your master/slave relationship then is primarily sexual?

No, I would say not. The relationship I share with my slave is very much mental as well as physical. It is becoming more and more encompassing, much deeper. We've come to various understandings about ourselves, our needs, and what we can and can not give, what we can ask of each other, what we hope to find in each other in a total relationship.

We often think of being master as being synonymous with being a sadist. Is that true for you?

I would say in my particular experience, yes. Certainly inflicting pain excites me. It's easy for me to punish him as well.

How do you punish your slave?

It depends on why I'm punishing him. What it is he's done that I've felt he needed to be punished for. Sometimes a paddle, sometimes a whip.

Do you ever inflict pain on him for other than punishment?

Yes, I do, for my own pleasure. It excites me, it turns me on. Part of the responsibility of owning a slave is to use that slave for your pleasure. Any master who has regular sanity has his own limits which he imposes on the relationship, physically and mentally. There are certain things that I would not do. Permanent damage, for instance, is something I'm not interested in inflicting on a slave.

Are you interested in marking them as your own?

With a chain collar and lock. I've considered branding, but I have not done it. The reason is that there's more visibility with the collar and lock. And that seems to satisfy me.

How did you go about getting a slave?

He came to me, and then there was a process. I don't believe that lasting relationships are found automatically. To me it's not enough to say he turned me on and the sex was good. It has to be more than just that. For a person to be a slave he has to be able to give himself up totally.

The master gives himself into the relationship as much as the slave does, though the intensity is somewhat different.

What does it feel like to own someone?

It's a challenge. Owning somebody is taking the responsibility to train them, to make them what you want them to be while letting them be what they have to be; letting them experience their own growth, while you grow.

I know one young man who wanted to be a part time slave. We had several good experiences, and I saw a lot of him for a short time. Then he decided that he wanted to be somebody's master. He thought he fell in love with a young man, a bottom whom he really desired. He called me about a month after that affair and, well, it had ended. He guessed he just wasn't ready for that kind of responsibility. He didn't realize how difficult it was to be master, to take that responsibility for a relationship and for someone else's life.

How do you act toward your slave? What kind of role do you move into?

I actually try to not move into a role. The feelings that I feel as a master are the same kind that I feel every day in most of my relationships. Certainly the master/slave relationship is a different branch, but the attitude is the same. I don't go into some kind of character to play master. As master, I act upon many more desires, ones that in normal society I may not do, but I don't feel like I go through any significant changes.

You are comfortable with things not done "in normal society." But beyond that, I know for instance that your slave does housekeeping for you and laundry. How do you feel comfortable with that?

The gift the slave gives is service, and that is simply one of many services that a slave can provide. Again, we're getting back to what I consider a difference between a bottom and a slave. A bottom may be someone that I play with who likes certain things, either physical or mental, certain kinds of dominant behavior from me, but I wouldn't necessarily, outside of the bedroom, say to that person, "Scrub my floor. Now, dump my trash. Now, do my laundry."

A slave is more complete than what we normally just call a bottom. A good slave gives everything he can.

I imagine that some people might think that you are selfish and arrogant.

Probably so. I'm fairly selfish, certainly. The experience that I have as a master with my slaves is that their joy is in serving. If there is no specific thing to serve, no dominance in the ways to serve, then they are very much "at sea."

What aspects of being a master satisfy you most? Least?

What satisfies me the most, I think, is the domination, the control.

The least? That's difficult to say. Basically I'm so comfortable with the relationship I have that there are really no major things that make me unhappy, other than the fact that logistically it's not very practical for us to live together.

Has having a slave changed your life?

It's made it better. Certainly it's fulfilled a need that I have that wasn't fulfilled before. We all search for various kinds of relationships, and that one seems to have been fulfilled for me.

What kind of advice would you give to someone who said they wanted to be a master?

Understand the responsibility. Understand the depth of the relationship. Try to understand whether or not the person who wants to be your slave is just a bottom, or just curious, or whether or not they are willing to make that kind of commitment. When a person becomes a slave, he really gives himself up to a master. Slavery is not a part-time kind of thing. Either you're someone's slave, or you're not. It's hard for most people to make that kind of major commitment. People really have to be in the right space to make it, to say, "Here I am. Take me. Do with me as you will."

Likewise understand yourself. Do you really want to be master? Can you make that kind of commitment to yourself? Will you be able to say "I'm a sadist" or to give orders simply because you want to? Go ahead. Find out. Any bottom will tell you there aren't enough masters to go around. You might as well be in control as anyone else.

Chapter 19

SLAVERY—NOW THAT SAYS IT ALL!

Robert Payne's book, *The Exchange* (Alternate Publishing, Forestville, CA, 1992) is an erotic, highly intense account of men bought and sold to give pleasure (sexual and otherwise) to their masters. It is the ultimate dominance/submission fantasy, the stuff of hard core leather relationships. It is fiction, pleasure-delivering, one-handed fiction, but fiction none the less. At least I think that it is. Some day "The Exchange," "The Network," or some other "Sex Slaves for Sale Group" may make itself known to me, but until then the idea will remain fiction.

To one degree or another, however, this fiction is the basic leather fantasy. For some it is a quest. For a few, this quest is accomplished. Slavery with a sexual orientation is no fiction. Men and women experience it.

I'll quickly grant that such a lifestyle attracts many more perpetual wanna-be's than people actually willing to adventure into the experience. In his *Leatherman's Handbook*, Larry Townsend writes about masters and slaves. His definition of the slave calls for total submission, a stay-at-home-and-obey attitude completely controlled by the omnipresent, omni-controlling top. Practically, such intensity is hard to come by, and even more difficult to sustain.

But there is a happy middle ground here: the lifestyle of

the part time submissive.

I'm not going to define what is ideal in the master/slave scene. There are those who have it defined to the point of a highly structured contract. I've read several slave contracts, and even wrote one once. My outlook, though, is that any relationship (including master and slave) is best defined by those in it. Simply put, what the master gets is only what the slave is willing to give. We're not talking about forced submission, kidnapping, violence, or abduction. What we call "slavery" is voluntary servitude: the attitude and ability of one person to surrender him/herself to the dominating will of another.

The primary ingredient in such an arrangement of course is the bottom's ability to let go of self-control, surrendering into the power of one who has the ability and desire to take temporary control. In the more serious aspects, masters move into a kind of ownership, as submissives surrender plans, time, and talents to service to the desires of the dominant.

Early on in such a relationship, the service rendered is usually sexual in nature. As the relationship develops the slave will most likely move into areas of service beyond fucking and sucking. The service will come to include housekeeping and gardening chores, surrender of finances, a matching of the slave's will to the desire of the master.

Lynn owns Jim. At first sight they appear as two handsome men in their early forties, friends and drinking buddies, maybe fuck buddies, but perhaps not. On closer observation, Jim wears a silver chain around his neck. It's heavier than most jewelry and is held in place by a small brass lock. Lynn has the key. The chain has been in place since Lynn took Jim as his slave. It was a quiet event, late one night after they had known each other about ten weeks.

Jim knew that Lynn had bought the chain, he wanted to be Lynn's "best boy."

When you hear Jim talk about it, you can tell he's happy. Lynn accepts Jim's service as his due, knowing that the relationship satisfies both of them. He enjoys the idea of owning another man, and finds pleasure in the obedience that Jim gives. Lynn tells Jim when to report and when to go, what to clean, what to wear, where to sleep. He finds pleasure in his slave's body in many ways: satisfying his lust, his sadism, his need to control, and his desire for pleasure.

Jim's pleasure is found in the pleasure he gives his master. As slave, he enjoys feelings of surrender that are devoid of stress, and without concern for decision making. He finds fulfillment, release, and a kind of communion in the worship of his master's body, and obedience to his master's will. There is satisfaction in being able to perform to his master's high expectations, a feeling of accomplishment in being able to take everything that Lynn dishes out to him.

There is intense pleasure in the way Lynn affects Jim physically. His control of his slave's body eventually brings orgasm. On other levels they have developed bonds of mutual awareness and psychic energy exchanges that are rarely found between two people. These phenomena are derived from the intense bonding that has taken place.

Actual master/slave relationships span a wide spectrum of definitions: the slave who pays a dominatrix for the opportunity to worship; the heterosexual pairings found in some of the many SM clubs and organizations; the male/male and female/female partners found clad in black leather on a Saturday night. Many are short lived, one night stands; others grow into long-term committed relationships.

95

If and when "The Exchange" invites me to an auction, I'll do my best to bring enough cash to get the man of my dreams. Short of that, at least the fantasy makes good reading.

Chapter 20

HOW TO BE YOUR MASTER'S BEST BOY

Slavery is only one expression of a leather lifestyle. Nevertheless, if you are to be a master, you're going to have to have an idea of what you want in a slave. I'm a firm believer that the definition of a slave's role is up to the master. Any "master" who allows his slave to set the definitions of his slavery is not a master. He or she may be a damn good top, but topping isn't mastering.

How you define your slave's (or slaves') service to you is up to you. Have confidence in what you want and work to get it. When you find it, cherish it because "best boys" are a true delight.

In hopes of guiding a few masters into expanding, by their control, a fine class of servants, I'm going to give out some advice. Concrete descriptions and exact rules depend upon the will of the master. So follow my suggestions as you desire. After all, only you can decide whom you're going to name "best boy." If you grant that I am experienced enough to be authoritative on the subject of master/slave relationships, then read on. Here you have "Jack's Rules for Slaves," guaranteed to make him or her "best boy," at least in my bedroom.

1. Say "Sir."

A substantial part of any human relationship entails speech. So have your slave(s) use the desired title

97

frequently and respectfully. You may prefer master, mistress, lord, milady, or even that he or she use your first name. What you are called depends upon your instructions. What they say is important, how they say it is essential.

Instruct them to use their voice to show deference, respect, and submission. Less speech is better than more. Sincerity is required. Without honesty and candor, they will never be "best."

2. Be zealous to please.

To give pleasure is the only reason for a slave to be in the master's presence. How they give pleasure will be defined by your instructions. How well they give pleasure will be determined by their attitude. A slave pleases by obedience, conformance to expectations, and by his/her approach to a master. Once a slave knows to do something, he should do it without having to be told. They should anticipate, within your guidelines, your wishes and do their best to do them well.

3. Surrender yourself as a gift.

What we're exploring, experiencing here if you will, is the creation of a polarity that can elicit incredible mental states, intense physical sensations, and strong bonding. A slave's willingness, surrender, and commitment are needed to bring "success" to your relationship. At stake is the co-creation of a unique relationship.

While the master "creates" the slave, the slave simultaneously creates the master. After all, how can anyone be dominant unless someone submits?

4.. Open yourself and become vulnerable to your master's will.

That, of course, is easier said than done. Our natural (?) reaction is to cover ourselves, to hide and protect ourselves. We have been taught to compete and assert. In this, slavery is a strong renunciation of worldly values, a serious affront to the status quo. It doesn't gain the usual benefits. Happily, other, more sublime victories, are to be had by submitting.

It is difficult to drop the defenses, the desires, the ego-tripping facades that we use to face the world each day. But the true slave finds solace in the master's will. Frankly, for the real slave in the right relationship, this is an incredible release, the experience of which is an immense reservoir of peace and calm. Best boys learn to enter this state.

5. Relax and accept your condition.

This is the art of letting go. Does the whip hurt too much? Is the slave jealous that you're paying attention to someone else? Are they bothered by your demands? Help them to let go. Encourage them to embrace their state as a chosen condition. Does it hurt? Teach them it's "OK" to feel it, to surrender to it, let it move them. Does it give him or her pleasure? Let them enjoy it, accept it, let it "take" them.

There is one important qualification here: Instruct your slaves that if they feel that the experience is dangerous to their health, they are to inform you immediately. Best boys need to be kept in the best physical condition. They need to accept pain, but not injury. There is a difference!

6. Study.

Your slaves should learn what turns you on. Give them time to work to improve their technique, whether it be folding laundry or sucking your cock. Let them know how you like them to act in public, in bed, at your feet. Show them how to fine tune their physical attention to your body. Help them learn how to give massages, how to make coffee, how to worship your body with every part of their body.

7. Respond.

Slaves should react to your attention. Some masters like to hear their slaves cry, see them squirm, feel them having orgasms. Others prefer quiet surrender. Let them know what kind of responses most please you, and encourage them to act accordingly.

Some responses can be spontaneous. Others can be planned. As it is feasible, there are a host of things slaves can do to show their submission to you. Invitations to dinner, bringing flowers or favorite foods, going "beyond the call of duty" in housekeeping or gardening are things they can do to show their responses. Give them "room" to communicate to you by word and deed. Help them to make you proud of them at all times.

8. Love your master.

I've saved the most important for last: Love will come naturally if it is to come at all. I'm not talking about being in love, I mean rather the decision your slave makes to prefer you, to see you as the center of his or her devotion and attention. Be the kind of master that will allow them to focus on you as a partner in this unique creation.

As master, be responsible for directing and maintaining the relationship. For your slave's part, let them take responsibility for serving you. Accept that service as your due and their pleasure. In that way, you will have the pleasure of having them be "best."

Chapter 21

REALITY THERAPY

I readily admit to being an idealist. I still search the classifieds looking for the boy of my dreams, expect that the next SM scene will send me into seventh heaven, and that after I have my next orgasm all my bills will have been mysteriously paid in full.

As of the writing of this book, though, I have grey hair and years enough of experience to know that for some "God only knows" reason we live on a less than perfect planet. I hope that this chapter can be short and sweet, but I'd be less of an author if I didn't include a bit of reality therapy in my book.

The message really is short and sweet. OK, it's not really sweet, but short. You will find a major discrepancy between your fantasy/expectations and what happens in real life. The person "in person" is going to look different than his or her picture, and probably be ten pounds heavier. There are going to be as many boring people at that leather workshop as you find anywhere else. That ideal slave will do everything except the dishes, be at your place on time, and miss his favorite television program, to say the least. You will be stood up, told you won't do, asked to stop before you've really started, and find yourself more often than not working hard to please a bottom.

Dungeons need cleaning. Toys have to be sanitized and put away. Crabs and scabies will walk down your leg.

Your search for a slave will take longer than you think, will involve innumerable phone calls leading to very few visits, and the repeatedly "best prospect" will stop returning your phone calls right after you decide that he is the one you want to own forever.

So take a deep breath and remember that this is planet earth. Sorry. If you've read this far, you're past the point of getting a refund!

I say all this not to discourage you, but to put things in perspective. Fantasy fulfillment takes work. Work, in this context, means being clear about what you want, committing yourself to accomplishing it, and persevering until you do. It means that you're willing to spend time, effort, and finances to find the right person, attract him or her, and negotiate the relationship you both want.

Getting the relationship you seek is no easy matter. Finding the "right" partner seems to take forever, and once you are over that hurdle, the process has only just begun.

Even the best trained, most experienced slaves need to be taught the unique demands that a new master has for his/her slaves. And, if you are new at this, the list of things *you* have to learn can seem endless.

Becoming the master you want to be takes a willingness to change. That may seem easy enough. But what we forget is that the changes might not be the kind we want to embrace. As an example, as a master you may want to work out every other day to build a muscular frame on your cute, young body. That fantasy may demand you eat a better breakfast, drink less alcohol, and be asleep an hour earlier than usual. Can you do it?

Mastery conjures up all sorts of thoughts about erotic activities, sexual adventures, and multiple orgasms. We think that it's all bondage, discipline, sucking, fucking, and body worship. But in reality, most of the time a master and slave spend together has little to do with those activities. You'll be surprised at how much time a slave spends simply waiting. Can you handle it?

Can you handle the responsibility itself? Are you willing to pay that much attention to one person? The first half hour with your new slave will most likely be a torrent of instructions. You'll find it all very exciting at first. But can you last more than a night? More than a week? A month? Will you still want this slave three months from now? The thrill of it all will wear away. If it's a game to you, the game will become very boring. You'll find that you've given him or her all of your time and now you have none for yourself.

It sounds as if I'm down on the whole idea of ever realizing your dream. I'm not. If a slave is what you seek, then go for it. Just go for it slowly. You really can't do it any other way anyway. It takes time to develop the levels of trust that dominance and submission require. And I will be the first to tell you not to get a slave who can't trust you.

It will be a matter of "getting to know you." Your new slave will want to know what you're thinking, how you're feeling, what turns you on and what turns you off. He'll expect you to be honest and open. He'll want to get into your head, to understand your expectations, your limits, your history.

Both of you will bring a lifetime of experiences into your first encounter. Is he or she here out of desperation? Curiosity? Love? Anger? Self-hate? Is he bouncing from a broken affair or convinced that he was born to serve you? I don't think it's necessary for you to have answers to these questions right now. But in time you will have to face why you're doing this, and how badly you want to do it. What will be in it for you? What do you want to be in it?

If the relationship is to last past the first disagreement, you'll have to have solid reasons for keeping this slave. Either having him is sufficient and has its own rewards, or you'll look to find someone else, or you'll give up your master fantasy entirely. Only time will tell. I always encourage wanna-be's to try out their fantasies. So, "go for it."

A while ago, I answered a classified ad from a guy who wanted a permanent master. When we talked on the phone he pleaded with me to give him a chance. I did. We met and I began my usual routine of ordering him around. It took less than fifteen minutes for him to say, "I'm sorry. This isn't for me." He was dressed and out the door within three minutes, muttering his apologies. He had literally driven 50 miles for 18 minutes of experience. I'm sorry to say, I think he thinks he failed. But he didn't. In fact, he learned. He may not have liked what he learned, but he learned all the same.

The simple, sad fact is that it's more difficult to live our fantasies than we know. Making our great idea real takes effort, patience, perseverance, trial and error. I've found that we've got to explore the dream on its own terms, letting it do its work of inner transformation and serious change, even as we let the dream itself change. It's a matter of letting go of our expectations of how the dream will be, and letting it have a life of its own.

We all have dreams, ideas, ideals. The particulars change, the details are different, but the process: think, attempt, learn, grow, think some more, and try again, is universal. Go for it, whatever it is, and may you have all the luck in the world. If you are willing to grow, you will have "all the luck in the world." The dream will help you create your own luck, which, of course, is where luck comes from in the first place.

Chapter 22

ROPES, WHIPS, AND OTHER DANGERS

Safe, sane, and consensual are the hallmarks of any leather activity. Today we most often think of safe sex as taking precautions against the spread of AIDS, and well we should. But there are a lot of other things of which we need to be mindful. Happily, leather play can be both safe and fun. With just a slight amount of effort, we can fulfill all sorts of fantasies without harm. The key, of course, lies in having the right information, taking precautions, and using common sense. In the final analysis, you are responsible for your health and safety. Play accordingly.

I will not pontificate as to what is safe activity between two consenting adults. I trust that you're an adult and will act in a responsible manner. Acting in a responsible manner means that you are informed. As in a court of law, ignorance is no excuse. Face the facts as outlined by your physician and follow them. We've heard it before, but it bears repeating: Don't allow another's bodily fluid (especially blood or semen) to come into contact with any open membrane in your body, i.e. mouth, rectum, vagina, eyes, cut, or wound.

I'm sure there are those out there who hate rubbers (condoms) as much as I do, but the inconvenience is well worth the reward. Sex is wonderful, but as the posters and ads say, "It's not worth dying for."

Happily, HIV is a lot less virulent than many think. Don't make it an excuse to cut yourself off (so to speak) from the pleasures your body can give and receive from others. With the right information you can learn to enjoy sex and stay healthy. There are many sexually active men and women who are still free of the AIDS virus. They stay that way by playing safely. HIV doesn't need spell the end of sex, only the end of unsafe sex!

But there are risks other than HIV. Several other STDs are in fact easier to catch. Though they may not be as deadly, they ought to be avoided.

Leather activity need not be dangerous. In fact, many leather activities offer a high degree of erotic stimulation without any risk of disease. There is no transfer of body fluids in healthy tit work, or cock and ball torture. Understanding and adhering to the need for cleanliness in one's toys (dildoes, whips, paddles, clamps, etc.) opens up a wide variety of safe activities. A good spanking with a clean clothes brush won't give you the clap. But there are other guidelines the CDC doesn't list. Tops and bottoms alike need to take responsibility for their safety and the safety of their partners. In any scene the top needs to insure that the bottom's skin isn't accidentally broken with welts or cuts, that his or her circulation isn't impeded by ropes or restraints. Check frequently that extremities (hands and feet) don't get cold or fall asleep. And being aware isn't only the top's responsibility. Bottoms ought not to be so "macho" as to endure health-threatening domination. Tell your slaves not to be afraid to ask you to stop. After all, you can't feel the effects as well as they can.

Often leather partners will choose a "safe word" for the bottom to signal the top that there is some kind of danger or that the bottom's limits are being unwisely exceeded.

There is no disgrace in asking for the scene to stop when one's health is endangered. Submitting oneself to danger is not "being a good slave," it is stupid.

In that regard, care should be taken with the use of hand cuffs as they are apt to cut off circulation. Tie those bottoms up well, but carefully. I always tie my knots in loops so that a quick pull on the short end loosens it.

Put your slaves in positions that they can maintain, and use padded restraints.

Equipment ought to be clean and some things (like dildoes and butt plugs) should never be shared without being decontaminated between uses. Make it a strictly "BYO" affair. Chlorine bleach (diluted in water in a one to ten solution) does wonders on dildoes. Soap and water never hurt anyone—at least that's what my mom taught me.

Since I'm in a "do and don't" kind of mood, do use lubricants with nonoxynol-9. If there is any amount of anal or vaginal play, be sure your fingernails are well trimmed and wear latex gloves. They can be bought in a box of 100 for under ten dollars. Use them once and throw them away. Remember: "No glove, no love".

If the taste of latex leaves something to be desired, use a flavored lubricant, and load on the nonoxynol-9 after the oral play and before insertion. You can also play well with chocolate, maple syrup, and whipped cream.

Avail yourself of good information. Ask your physician, and read any (or all) of the many guides to safe sex. Attend informational meetings put on by leather clubs and health organizations. I can't show you knots, or teach techniques in the pages of this book, so avail yourself of expertise in other ways. Remember that the only stupid question is the one that isn't asked. After all, it's your health and that of your partners that matter.

I'd rather avoid the subject of drug use, but if we are to play safely, we must understand the dangers posed by it. First off, I am a libertarian, a hedonist, and a stubborn individualist. I don't like people telling me what to do. I suspect you feel much the same way. Secondly, I don't want to be hypocritical, and sound as if I'm a teetotaler, abstainer, or prude. Thirdly, the laws of the land concerning regulated pharmaceuticals are not a subject germane to this book.

There are substances, both legal and illegal, that need to be considered in the SM sub-culture, not because you ought not to use them, but because you will run into their use. To do so in this decade all you need to do is go to grammar school!

I'm free-wheeling and easy going. I enjoy a relaxing drink once in a while. I'm not going to tell you to abstain, but I will emphasize that you need to take care. Prohibition didn't work, and caused more social ills than it solved. Our current drug laws have created the same kind of shoot-em dead mentality as well. The simple fact remains though that what is illegal needs to be avoided. There is no use in getting yourself, or your partners, into any trouble that has a jail sentence attached to it. Be smart, play clean and sober.

Legality, though, is the least of the reasons to abstain from perception-altering liquids, pills, powders, and smokes. Good SM is a mind-altering trip. There is no advantage to doubly altering one's mind.

My experience is that the use of drugs, in the long run, will diminish, if not end, a good SM scene. Relationships built around drug (ab)use won't do well either.

Tops especially need to stay in control. That control is not only directed towards their bottoms and slaves. They also need to stay in control of themselves. I suppose that's why I don't like to get drunk. I don't like to lose control! There is the tendency, of course, on the part of the slave to want to use drugs such as poppers, grass, coke, booze, etc., to lessen the effect of the pain to which he or she might be subject. I understand that wish very well. Truth is there's nothing as helpful as a sniff of amyl to help one endure a pair of bare metal alligator clips on one's nipples. But what happens is that the slave feels the pain less, even as it does its possibly destructive job. In order to avoid injury, the slave needs to feel the intensity as it affects the body so he can tell the top what is really being felt. If the bottom loses his ability to feel, he loses his ability to communicate what is happening. The result is that both the top and the bottom cease dealing with reality, and injury becomes more likely.

Drugs alter perceptions and outlooks as well. More often than not, depending on the kind of drug being used, even moderate drug use will slow down the scene. Before you know it, you might both be asleep. But that is certainly not the only possible effect. I find, for instance, that coke causes its users to become irritable, even mean. One mild-mannered bottom got persistent to the point of obnoxiousness when sniffing coke. This is not a good way to have a scene.

SM is going to change things enough by itself, the addition of drugs is only going to compound the situation, not make it better. Enough said. Play all you want, but do it safely. As the wonderful nurse at our local clinic told me after my last check up: "Honey, I don't know what you're doing, but keep on doing it." Little did she know how glad I was to get permission!

Chapter 23

SCENES THAT GO WRONG

I'm sure that I'm not the first to tell you that we live in an imperfect world, or, at best, one where things don't always go the way we think they ought. This is no reason, however, to lie down and die. It just means that we need to be prepared for something less than the best.

My friends marvel at the kinds of risks I take. Face it, I got a good deal of my education in leather because I was willing to take chances. I never really knew if the guy I was going home with was trustworthy, if it was safe to be walking those downtown streets, or if I'd get myself in more trouble than I could handle.

Fact is, I marvel that after all these years, I can count my "bad" experiences on one hand and none of them were really that bad. I credit my fortune to a guardian angel that works overtime. Even angels can be over-worked and the un-wished for comes true. Yes, scenes may go wrong.

The best way to get out of a scene that's going wrong is to insure that you don't get into it in the first place. Prevention and caution are habits that all tops ought to form early on, not to mention that those are habits their bottoms need to start with as well. It's a matter of common sense. Now, don't go ruining your good time by confusing common sense with paranoia, insecurity, or an irrational demand that everything be perfect. Instead weigh your risk-taking against the gains and the good times.

The first rule of safety is to keep yourself in a position where you can control yourself. I can write that because I'm presuming that you are masterful in your relationships and desire to stay in control. If you happen to be a bottom, then the first rule is going to be to keep yourself in a position where you can trust that the person in control can be trusted.

Yes, accidents occur. The trick is to minimize their occurrences and to lessen their effect. That's done by knowing your partner, your equipment, and your play space.

I'm not big on rules but there are some that are both obvious and imperative: play safely, use condoms and gloves, and stay away from intoxicants and pharmaceuticals. Discuss the scene before you begin and know your mutually agreed upon limits. Most importantly, know with whom you are playing. That doesn't mean you can't play with strangers. You can, but your play needs to be moderated by the depth of intimacy you share. The better you know each other, the higher the level of trust you can have, and therefore the greater the intensity that can be aroused.

If something feels strange, either before or during a scene, take the care necessary to find out why you feel as you do. Not everyone goes into SM with the same pure motives (grin) and not everyone is as healthy, either physically or mentally, as they appear. I'll be quick to add that the number of "crazies" you'll meet is wonderfully low and the dangers aren't anywhere near as great as the uninitiated dread. Common sense is still the rule.

If, for whatever reason, things do go wrong, take quick and decisive action. Stay calm, and assure your bottom that you are doing everything you can as fast as you can to remedy the situation. This is where preparation is essential. For instance, the scissors you have handy will end the bondage a lot more quickly than trying to untie ropes. Aren't you glad they were handy?

If the emergency is physical, take physical measures to correct it, such as stopping the scene, getting the bottom to rest, or calling for emergency help. Have those phone numbers handy.

The probability is greater that the emergency will be of an emotional nature. I remember a wonderful bottom named Lou, who broke down in tears during a scene. He was remembering an abusive childhood spent in an orphanage and a father who left his mother before he was born. It was a stressful remembrance for him. Though we didn't end the scene, I did take time to listen, to encourage, and to comfort. The pause allowed him to regain his composure and his desire to play. Then we continued.

SM arouses all sorts of intense emotions. Again, be prepared for their appearance and use care and common sense to deal with them. Keep yourself in control and use that control to lead your bottom into a space where the conflict he or she may be feeling can be assuaged.

The same goes for yourself as well. If you feel yourself losing control, getting angry, nauseated, or tired, be masterful enough to do what's necessary. Stop, rest, reflect, and act prudently. You are in charge, make good decisions, even if it means ending the scene. Believe me, there'll be a lot more scenes later if you play smart now.

An SM scene is no place for therapy. There is the chance that eventually you will be playing with someone who needs professional help. Recognize what is appropriate for an SM scene, and what isn't. Whips and chains are not instruments to use with bravado. Simply put, know yourself and your partner. Stay cool and get help if necessary. Chances are that your scenes will never go wrong. The best way to make sure that is the case is to plan ahead. Boy scouts know what they're talking about when they say "Be prepared." Whether you're scouting for boys or girls, follow that advice.

Chapter 24

WHAT'S IN A
TOP'S TOY BAG?

Having collected leather toys for more years than I care to tell, I've garnered quite a usable assortment. I'd like to give you a tour of my tools.

The first thing to notice is that I keep my toys, at least those of them that will fit, in a gym bag. I was once told to buy myself a leather bag for my equipment, but I've never quite had the extra dollars to do so. (If any admiring reader wants a gift idea, there's one.) On the other hand, the fact that it's only a nylon gym bag means that I can ride on public transportation with it, and it's lightweight. It doesn't look very threatening.

The first two items are easy to come by: rope and clothespins. I keep small items like clothespins and rawhide laces in their own plastic zip-lock bags so they're easily accessible. I keep dildoes in bags as well, to assure they stay clean and safe. Twenty to thirty clothespins are sufficient for most scenes. Actually you'll probably only use two, four or six at a time anyway. Wash the rope before using it, thereby making it softer and easier to manipulate. It's a good idea to prevent its unraveling by dipping the ends in glue. You'll want ropes of different lengths. Some shorter (about 4 feet), others longer for more serious bondage like tying your bottom spread eagle to a mattress. I use rubber bands to keep the ropes neatly folded.

A pair of handcuffs is a natural as well, though I only use them for scene starters, since they often rub the skin and cut circulation.

Leather wrist and ankle restraints are much better, come in numerous styles, and pose much less danger. I made my first pair, and lined it with rabbit fur. Later I bought more substantial cuffs.

Have plastic wrap and duct tape handy for those special bondage scenes. A pair of scissors to release someone is important as well. If possible, get the kind used to cut off bandages, as they are shaped to slide under the bondage material without endangering the skin. On a similar note, a few lengths of ace bandage are very versatile. They make excellent blindfolds, ball stretchers and wrist/leg restraints.

Condoms and lubricant are important toys as well. In fact, they are so important you should never party without them.

One or two pairs of tit clamps are good for when the tit torture gets a bit more intense. I use the kind with rubber shields on their ends, though I have been known to slip the shields off as my bottom moved into the enjoyment of more intense pain.

In another plastic bag, I keep all sorts of small play things: shoe laces, leather thongs, ball stretchers, fishing weights, nylon fishing line, small hooks to attach the weights to the tit clamps.

As expensive and intricate as some toys can be, creativity can reduce their cost. For instance, two clothespins strung together with a piece of rawhide make very serviceable tit clamps. They're not expensive, and can easily hold those fishing weights.

Finding low cost equipment takes a bit of shopping.

Though most people buy a lot of leather equipment at a hardware store, don't forget craft stores, sewing centers, department stores, and pharmacies. I got a box of Texas catheters (penis sheaths with a nozzle on the end to which you can attach a plastic hose) at a pharmacy recently. I had to go to three places to find them. The most difficult task was asking the druggist about them. I found it embarrassing. If you shop in a gay neighborhood, the embarrassment level is greatly reduced.

Since we're on drug store selections, I have a small rubber syringe for giving enemas. And, of course, a plastic bag full of latex gloves. At home I also have a larger enema bag and a few syringes of commercially-prepared enemas. Some bottoms just don't know how to "show up clean." Again, this kind of equipment is used only once, or is thoroughly sanitized in bleach before every use.

My first and favorite instrument for discipline is a leather belt that I've had for about a dozen years. Since I often wear it when I go out, it's not officially "in the bag," but it is handy. Other tools for bun-warming include wooden and leather paddles, cats of nine tails, whips, riding crops, and brushes. Start with one or two small inexpensive items. Each will have its own feel and effect. I once had a discipline scene with a guy who had over 150 different "spanking toys." He had a paddle fetish, and had made—with great care and artistry—many of the wooden paddles I used on his ass. Kitchen utensils, rug beaters, bamboo, fancy canes, and various types of tree branches (hickory, willow, etc.) rounded out his collection.

You might have to make a trip out to the "burbs" to find some items. I bought a wonderful buggy whip at a riding supply store once. Such stores are not easy to find but are well worth the trip. Don't worry what the clerk thinks; you'll never see him or her again!

I keep four different dildoes in my bag. Always wash them with bleach, and never use them on more than one person between thorough cleaning! Covering them with a rubber helps make the cleaning easier and insures an even higher level of safety.

The first dildo is embarrassingly small, but the others are larger. Two others (much larger) I keep at home, and reserve for people who can take it. If you proceed slowly and gradually increase the size inserted, a rectum can expand quite nicely. I also have a butt plug. They're great for longer retention times.

I'm not really big on medicinal-type toys, but you may want to bring along a tube of Ben-Gay. I know a professional dominatrix who always brings a supply of anal-ease. She uses it to get her client's ass to relax. If your bottom has trouble taking what you're giving, that may make the scene easier, if you want to make it easier.

Every good bag should have a few candles and a pack of matches. Cheap candles burn at a lower temperature and cause less pain. Try them on yourself first so you know how to do it, and what effect they will have.

I keep an assortment of small locks in my bag as well. I have them locked onto a metal ring. In the same bag I have a set of keys. The locks are locked before I use them insuring that when I use them, I will first have to have the key handy to open them for use. Never use a lock unless you are positive, by having opened it right then and there, that you have the key.

I also have a dog's choke chain and several collars. Some are made to buckle on, some to lock on, one has wrist restraints attached to it. I also have a home-made leather blindfold.

Then of course, there's a leather hood. Mine is homemade, but the store bought varieties are probably better. They come with and without eye and mouth holes. They lace, zip, and/or buckle. The lace ones are more versatile in that they fit more sizes. Going up the price scale, there are wonderful leather body bags, lock-on mitts that render hands useless, body harnesses, full-body restraints, etc.

There are various chastity, penis, and vagina covering devices. Buy two pair, one for your bag and one for mine! For more specific apparatus, get yourself on a mail order list or visit a local adult book store.

Larger equipment won't fit into the bag. I'll leave a discussion of stocks, crosses, cages, etc., for the next chapter.

121

Chapter 25

SERIOUS LEATHER
AND LARGE TOYS

I've got to give my friend Mark credit for having the best basement in the Midwest. It's the size of a comfortable apartment and is absolutely loaded with toys. Sex toys, that is. The place could be a showroom for the best kink catalog in the industry. Truth is, Mark does sell the stuff and has the uncanny knack of being able to get most anything legal. So if I'm going to include in my list of toys too large to fit in a top's toy bag, all I have to do is reflect on his basement.

Where do I start in this mind-boggling arena? How about with a two ton hoist with either boot straps or boots bolted to a cross piece so that you can hang your submissive upside down?

There is the usual dog cage that fits two. How about a bed? If that's not enough then try his sling or obstetrician's examining table. He doesn't have a dentist's chair, but he does have a "table" with holes for roping your playmate down. The center drops out to expose the mid section of your bound slave for your pleasure.

There are (it seems) miles of tubing hooked to a vacuum pump as well as electrical devices such as violet wands, vibrators, low amperage generators, and a cattle prod. In the non-electrical area, there are tubes and containers for enemas and water (add wine, soap, catnip, but only if you know what you're doing). Needless to say, the walls are replete with smaller toys such as crops, whips, chains, ropes, hoods, handcuffs, as well as cast iron restraints for neck, wrists, ankles, wrists at the waist, wrist to thigh, and cages for the head. All of these are also available in leather as well.

On the far wall, to the right as you come down the stairs, is a unique restraint device, called an Amsterdam box. It is a shallow closet (2 feet deep at most). Its back wall has appropriately placed leather straps, to hold one's boy or girl tightly within the closet. It closes with a sliding door to make the bondage complete. Not to deprive a master of the use he or she may wish to make of the slave thus bound, there are small doors in the sliding door that may be used to gain access to the bound servant in the appropriate areas.

No dungeon is complete without a cross, so Mark has a St. Andrew's Cross. It is shaped liked an "X" and holds his chattel in a spread eagle position. Crosses also come in the traditional "T" shape.

For his annual party, Mark will assemble a full size (10x10) jail in his living room. The guy takes his SM seriously.

My favorite "large toy" is a "peg seat," a low stool or chair with a dildo firmly attached to the seat so that its occupant is happily but firmly impaled on it.

The list of furniture-sized accouterments can go on for pages, of course, with stocks, beams, posts, benches, chairs, etc. One's imagination can literally run wild.

And that is, in fact, how a good dungeon is put together. The peg seat mentioned above for instance is one of my home-made, not-so-expensive contraptions. I had read about peg seats in a book somewhere, and decided to make one for myself (or should I say for my slave's self?). One day while walking through a large department store, I saw a short stand used to support a seat in a motor boat. It was sturdy and had holes in the right places to bolt a seat to it. Cost: less than ten dollars.

I brought it home, cut a square piece of plywood, fastened the end of a broom handle in its center, then put the plywood in place on the base. It then only needed a few holes drilled in it so that I had places to fasten ropes for tying down nuts, and a few hooks in the side for attaching wrist restraints. Voila, the best seat in the house!

Ideas are really the basis of good SM, and good ideas spring from research, discussion, and observation. Visit the "sex toy" stores in your area, and patronize them as you can, but you don't always have to drop a bundle. A good harness, for instance, costs over 60 dollars. On the other hand, the parts for one cost less than fifteen. Borrow a book from the library about leather crafting, and you've got the genuine, home made version with an evening's work.

Read magazines and invest in the catalogs that are advertised. There are even a few good books (illustrated) that show these large devices. Some even give directions on how to make them. And don't limit your reading to modern, glossy brochures. A book on the history of punishment, for instance, will give rise to lots of great ideas. Those Puritans knew what they were doing.

When you "make your own," do so carefully. Test everything for strength and build it stronger than you think necessary. Try it out on yourself first to insure safety. Remember that big toys need to be cleaned just as carefully as small ones. I never use that peg seat for instance without putting a condom on the dildo. (Safe is the first word in the credo, "Safe, sane, and consensual.")

This talk about "large sex toys" makes me think about "large sex organs." But you knew that about me I'm sure! The largest and most important sex organ we have is our brain. Not only is that where we experience the thrill of the sensations, but that is where the ideas, the creativity, and the drive to realize them originates. The best scenes are well-planned. The best equipment comes from well thought-out ideas that are well executed.

There is more to SM than quick anonymous sex. The best leather encounters take time for planning and preparation. I once built a dungeon in the basement of a home I owned. After two years, there were still improvements to be made and new ideas to be put into practice. Fortunately, there is enjoyment in the getting ready as well as in the having done.

Safe, sane, and consensual mean that leatherfolk have to think. Thinking provides more than safety, though. It provides excitement, diversity, originality, satisfaction, and pleasure.

Chapter 26

DUNGEONS AND PLAYROOMS

An often stated fact about leathersex is that it takes preparation. Good scenes don't just happen. They happen because someone gathered the right equipment in the right place at the right time with the right people.

As soon as I wrote the previous sentence, I remembered one of my most memorable scenes. It was with my good friend John B. I had just met him at the RamRod on New York's lower West side. We went back to his room (he didn't even have his own apartment), and had a great time with my equipment. Equipment? Did I say equipment?

In reality we played with nothing more than my shoe laces, my belt, and each other. That was enough for our first scene, complete with bondage, discipline, and great sex.

At the other side of the spectrum you can spend thousands of dollars on clothes, toys, furniture, and the playroom. Send off for any SM catalog and you'll see what I mean. Slings, crosses, cages, stocks, and beds don't come cheap. Add a full assortment of restraints, chains, pulleys, ropes, whips, and paddles and you're on your way. Unless you're a professional dominant, none of it is tax deductible.

Play spaces and the things you put in them either add a great deal to the leathersex experience or detract a great deal. Only you (or your architect) can really design the area that fits your needs, your desires, and your situation. Begin by taking stock of where you are and what you have.

Don't be afraid to improvise and experiment. The only caution that I'll throw your way is to make sure that anything you build or buy is constructed to withstand the stresses you will subject it to. You don't want a chair or post collapsing under the weight of your slave. Use strong brackets, wood and metal that are sturdier than necessary, and manufacturing techniques that will withstand pressure and strain. Use strong bolts. Counter sink them. Use lock washers, industrial strength materials, and assemble carefully. Measure twice, cut precisely. If it's wrong, don't cut corners, do it again.

I know a guy who lost a testicle because the sling he was lying in broke away from the ceiling. Not a good move.

As with anything else, there's been a progression in the kinds of spaces where I've played. My early scenes were simply in a bed, with ropes attached to the bed posts or strung under the mattress. In those days I lived in a small two room apartment.

There wasn't room for much, but I did devise a bondage rack that bolted into the doorway between the bathroom and the bedroom. It was a simple frame of two by fours that fit into the door jambs and lintel. By placing a post on each side of the jambs and bolting them to each other, there was no need to nail or screw anything into the doorway itself. I then put a good number of eye bolts and hooks into the two by fours. You'll find you'll need and want a lot more of them than you first think, as you can never have enough. By surrounding my slave with eye bolts, I could effectively weave a rope web around him for some rather secure bondage.

Add to that the usual candle light and appropriate music and you have a space ready to enjoy your next encounter. When done, it all simply tucks into a closet and no one (except you and the slave) will ever know!

I went from one end of the spectrum to the other. I moved from that apartment into a home I had purchased nearby. Why did I choose that house? Because it had a vegetable cellar just begging to be transformed into a dungeon. Tucked in a corner of the basement, it was out of the way but never out of mind. It took a bit of cleaning and the application of numerous bolts and hooks here and there, but it was ideal.

My friends still talk about the good times in that space. It was only about nine by nine but it was just right. And what made it right? Well, I think it was care. When I write about dungeons and playrooms, I'm really talking about mood-setting and image-creating. Dimmed and indirect lighting, candles, lanterns, music, warmth, the absence of outside noises, carpets, cushions, pictures, and art all help create sights, sounds, and sensations that excite the mind.

We're back again to the sex organ of the brain, aren't we?

The way you present your dungeon should achieve two objectives. The first is utilitarian. Make it functional. Masters have their whips and paddles hanging on the wall to keep them neat and to keep them handy. The second reason is just as important. Seeing all those whips and paddles hanging there impresses the mind and sends signals. Examine the effect of mirrors, photos, sconces, spotlights, speakers, heaters. What is the availability of a place to relax, to clean up, to get intense?

My grandmother used to say that "Roma wasn't built at once." You'll find that improving your dungeon and

129

increasing your collection of equipment is an on-going pleasure. As I've said before, those catalogs will give you lots of ideas. Getting to know others into the SM scene will also help. They will introduce you to carpenters, metal workers, and SM experts who can give you good tips and help you solve difficult space problems.

If you don't see it, ask for it. Many of the catalogs and leather stores can help you find things you can't find by yourself.

You're going to find that, until you really do have a live-in slave, being a master is work. You're the one who's going to have to prepare the space and return it to useable condition when you're done.

And that's important.

Scenes aren't something you rush into if you want the maximum enjoyment. Check out your dungeon well in advance of your slave's arrival. Get the lights, the music, and the temperature right. You may not feel like doing it when he or she leaves, but remember to go back and return everything to its place. Clean and disinfect the equipment, as necessary.

I'm back in an apartment, so I don't have a dungeon right now. But if your experience is anything like mine, your dungeon is going to become a very special place. You'll go there to dream, to relax, to meditate, to commune with your inner self. It will become uniquely yours with an energy and power that reflects who and what you are. Have fun with it. Its rewards will be remarkable.

Chapter 27

ALL TIED UP AND EVERYWHERE TO GO

The most exciting things seem to happen the first time around. At least first times always excite me. My first SM scene centered around bondage.

For David, the same was true. We met at my apartment. He was 30 minutes late, and nervous as hell. Fact is, I thought he was going to be a no-show. You get a lot of that these days. (Seems no one pays attention to Misses Manners or Vanderbilt anymore.) But eventually the door buzzer signaled my date was here. I let him in, welcomed him, offered him a drink (which he declined), then we talked for most of an hour.

I once learned in a job interview that the more you let the other guy say, the more *he* will trust you. As time passed, David relaxed, shared his ideas and hopes, and looked more ready for his first encounter. As he sat in the easy chair, I walked over and put a pair of handcuffs on him. It was all part of my "Go slow" strategy.

I moved a wooden captain's chair into the middle of the living room, placing it just under a seldom-noticed hook in the ceiling. I asked David to sit in it. Once he was seated, I brought several lengths of rope from the bedroom. I wrapped a length around his chest and arms and across the back of the chair. Still fully clothed, he had reached the first stage of immobility.

131

Of course he could have stood up and taken the chair with him, but the best scenes are a slow progression. Little by little, the bondage, the lack of freedom, and the intensity of the situation would increase. I bound each of his ankles with leather restraints and chains. I pulled his feet back behind the chair and hooked the chains together. Now he couldn't stand if he wanted to.

I wrapped an ace bandage over his eyes. It was meant to help screen out the rest of the world. Instead it made him uncomfortable. He asked me to remove it, and I did.

Bondage trips really are wonderful. The end result is often a very relaxing and expansive feeling, but to get there one needs to feel good the whole time.

I turned on some classical music. I undid the handcuffs, replacing them with padded leather wrist restraints. I loosened the cord around his chest and began to remove his shirt. I don't think anyone had ever stripped him before.

Being tied hand and foot can have the effect of "allowing" a person to experience things they would otherwise resist. Having given me "permission" to tie him, David had also, unconsciously, given me permission to do more. It was a "more" he wanted to experience, but something that he was not willing to verbalize. The bondage let him accept it.

Once his shirt was off, I replaced the ropes, criss-crossing his chest, being careful to leave his nipples exposed. I tweaked them once or twice. I undid his belt.

Bondage is fun, but as in many SM scenes, it is a lot of work. Scenes with more advanced "bottoms" demand more elaborate tying schemes. The top must be constantly on the lookout for ropes that are too restrictive. That is, those that cut off the flow of blood. Cold hands or feet, or having an extremity fall asleep are sure signs that the bondage is not safe.

I always tie my knots in loops that can be quickly untied. One of the advantages to chains is that clips can be undone easily. Leather thongs, on the other hand, can be very difficult to undo, so they should be used with caution or with bandage shears nearby.

I undid David's leg restraints, to be able to pull off his pants and expose his genitals. Once that was accomplished, I re-tied his legs. I put a clothespin on each of his nipples. This would send endorphins through his blood stream, helping to give him a sense of euphoria.

Then my bondage became more intricate. I laced his cock and balls in leather thongs and used a "parachute" device to surround his testicles. From it I hung some weights. Immobile and helpless, but not un-protected, David began to drift.

I put a hood over his head. This one had eye holes so that he didn't mind it. The feel and smell of leather surrounded him.

I removed the clothespins, played with his nipples a bit and replaced the clamps in a slightly different position. I moved my body close to his face so that he could feel the hair on my chest.

It's not quite fair for me to presume what David felt. I am only guessing what he experienced. He was in a heightened state of passion, as amply demonstrated by his erection. He was breathing deeply but quietly, eyes closed. He appeared to be drifting.

There is a state one enters in the best of scenes. It feels like you are floating in space, far from the pull of gravity. The Universe surrounds you, and is lit by millions of distant points of light.

I experience such states. There is a strange and warm

sensation. I feel like I've entered an expansive dimension. At the same time, though, this Universe seems to be within. As expansive as it feels, it is not cold or lonely, but supportive and filled with energy. Often there is the sound of celestial music, a New Age symphony, an angelic chorus. It is the place of the heart.

But perhaps I personalize too much. The truth is that such scenes are always different, always the unique creation of the people in them. Have fun with whatever you create.

Chapter 28

NOW HERE'S A TOPIC!

SM is not a mindless passion or irrational impulse. It springs from deeply felt and very real needs, urges, and desires. Its fountain is the subconscious; its river bed, life. But all that academic sounding stuff can be a bit much. So let me just "get down and dirty". Let me write about spanking.

I've whipped a lot of ass in my leather career, and some of those scenes still amaze me. In fact, it was a session with a guy out in the suburbs that proved to me that I have limits—and I was the one doing the whipping! It didn't hurt me at all, but it was more than I could take.

Several years ago I wrote an "Application for Training to Serve a Master." In it I described three reasons for discipline—One: the master's pleasure. It can be exciting to whip an ass, thigh, or back. The harder the more exciting. Spanking, belting, and paddling are downright arousing. Two: Bottom's like it, or at least want it, or at least want to see if they can take it. Generally, bottoms have a desire for it and are satisfied, given pleasure by receiving it. Three: Some discipline is real punishment for the breaking of a "rule". This is corporal punishment to enforce discipline and states, in a physical and memorable way, that the master is in control. It underlines one's dominance and the other's submission. This third type of discipline is usually most painful, least used, and of short

The Master's Manual

duration. Having gotten it once, your slave won't want to break that rule again.

Before I go much further, let me define terms. The idea of discipline includes spanking (with one's hand or belt), paddling, whipping, strapping, birching, and caning. The tools can be wooden paddles like the ones used in fraternities, belts, whips, riding crops, wooden spoons, saplings such as "hickory sticks," leather straps and paddles, cats (whips that are bunches of leather thongs). They can be of various sizes, widths, and textures.

And the people who get paddled have all sorts of motives as well. Paul likes to take it through his spandex shorts, and doesn't want much sex with it. Give him a short drink of cheap brandy, then go at his ass for hours.

Art has an ass that's tough. He likes it BA (bare ass), and likes to know that he'll end up with welts.

Chuck, on the other hand, is into mutual scenes. He loves to "trade swats." Five on him and then five on you. "Take it like a man" is his attitude and his satisfaction.

A spanking scene can be mutual, strictly dominance and submission, or a part of a wider scenario.

The best effect (or so *they* tell me) comes from starting the action slowly, and slowly building in your effect. I often start a spanking scene by swatting the butt, still in its protective clothing, first with my hand, then gradually increase the severity of the instrument, the force of the application, and the speed of the administration. (Sounds erudite, doesn't it?)

Hit in various places, concentrating on a spot for a time and then aiming somewhere else. Take a short break and start over. Caress and kiss a red spot, feel the heat of the area, help the bottom to relax, then go to it again.

Physical intimacy is an important part of a spanking

136

scene. The domination can arouse deep affection on the bottom's part and he/she may likewise respond to softness with wild lust and unadulterated devotion.

Positions should vary as well. Have the bottom over your knee or tied spread eagle on the bed. I like to strap a guy down to a footrest in the living room, ass available. Restraints and gags help. Sometimes, though, it's just nice to let them hold you as you apply the pain.

The spanking fraternity is large, but discovering it isn't always easy. And it is more than a "fraternity," since it certainly includes women, both dominants and submissives. It crosses lines of sexual orientation, age, and lifestyle.

The book, *Male Fantasies/Gay Realities* by George Stambolian, has an interview with a masochist. Let me quote from his dialogue.

"How is the pain inflicted?

"With a wide leather belt. I can take it to a point where I think I can't take it any more, and then I can switch it off. I seem to have no feeling.

"Like some mystics you've learned to master your body through your mind.

"Yes, I have done that.

"You do this because it gives him pleasure, and because you prove your . . .

" . . . masculinity.

"To him and you yourself?

"Yes, to both of us"

And later he continues:

"I have a man now who can look at me and get excited. It turns me on, and I'll do anything for that feeling, to keep it. And I want him to beat me harder because I don't want him to look anywhere else to find that satisfaction. And that's answering the question about pain and pleasure. I'm

taking my pain because I'm getting pleasure out of it."
Whether your "end" is giving cr receiving, enjoy—that's
what leather is all about.

Chapter 29

SPARE THE ROD, SPOIL THE SLAVE?

There are significant differences between corporal punishment and the infliction of pain for the giving of pleasure: technique, reason, and effect come to mind right away.

A person can endure a significant amount of pain from a whip, strap, hand, or paddle if their application begins slowly and builds to a higher, faster, and stronger level. This technique is used when the spanking or whipping is meant to give pleasure to either partner. Warming an ass prepares it for heavier discipline as the body adjusts itself to increasingly higher levels of pain. When the discipline begins at a higher level of intensity, the pain is much more difficult to tolerate.

During the times that pleasure is the reason for the spanking, there is (usually) a warmth, camaraderie, and intimacy that is lacking when the punishment is for the sake of punishment. At such times, caressing, kissing, foundling, and stroking are often intermixed with the application of pain.

And lastly, discipline feels different and effects a slave or bottom differently. Whereas many bottoms enjoy a paddling, most will do their best to avoid the paddle when it is applied as a punishment. Strange as it may seem, the purpose and technique create a wholly different experience when the top wields a whip as a means of correction or penance.

Many novices (and some not so new to the scene) think that both forms of discipline are the same—but they aren't. Discipline is a significant tool in a master's repertoire, but it is one that is often misunderstood and misapplied.

Real discipline "works" best in relationships that have continuity to them. It is meant to alter behavior. That doesn't mean that paddling and such can't be part of a short term scene. They certainly can be, though intense discipline demands a level of trust not easily reached in a fleeting encounter. The making and breaking of rules, and subsequent "punishment" are often part of the role-playing that occurs in SM encounters. I'm not going to presume to tell two (or more) people what should happen in their SM scene, but such discipline has a different flavor to it.

Some tops impose rules during a scene in order to create a reason for punishment. Likewise, some bottoms break the rules in order to "force" the top to punish them. In either case, if the scene works, then it is right for its participants. But all too often such artificiality is uncalled for. The simple recognition of rights and reasons can eliminate the need for such play-acting entirely.

What I mean is this: if a top wants to spank, paddle, whip, or otherwise warm up his bottom's bottom he doesn't need to use rules to gain "permission" to do so. As the dominant partner with a consenting bottom, he already has that permission. The top's pleasure is reason enough to proceed. In a real master/slave relationship, the top is in control and that is basis enough for him or her to do as s/he feels, within the limits of sanity, safety, and consent. But the vast majority of leather scenes never approach the intensity of a true master/slave relationship. Most of the

140

time, the leather scene is simply an acting out of fantasy. The scene is kept in the realm of play, and is seldom, if ever, allowed to affect one's life and lifestyle. That's the way life is, and it's liable to stay that way for a long time to come.

The problem with imposing rules in order that they be broken, or breaking rules simply for eliciting discipline is that both cases set up a scenario for failure.

At a "Novice Night" I was asked about a top who piled rules upon rules in order to make his bottom break them. It seemed he wanted to force the bottom to deserve a punishment. The bottom, for his part, found it frustrating, since his intention was to please his "master," an unattainable goal since the rules were impossible to keep. The bottom would have been very happy to please his master by receiving the discipline. There was no need to force it on him. He was willing to endure it for his master's pleasure. Instead, he felt a strong sense of failure since he couldn't keep all the rules his master had imposed.

As Lynn, an experienced master says, "You don't need to break a rule for me to punish you. I'll do it just because I want to do it. If you want a paddling, don't fuck up, just ask me for it, and you'll get it." Lynn can speak that way because of his own self-confidence. He recognizes the rights and responsibilities inherent in an SM relationship, and is comfortable with the gratifications they offer.

The best SM scenes are learning experiences. Discipline is a useful and necessary tool. With it a master can teach his slave how to behave, and help him modify his behavior to give greater pleasure to his master. Early on in their relationship, Jim, Lynn's slave, often came prematurely, much to his master's displeasure. The application of a heavy black belt across Jim's ass cured that habit very quickly.

Discipline is a necessary part of domination. It is a valuable tool for transforming a slave's actions and attitude. Though it ought not to be administered in anger, it needs to be intense enough to get the message across with some feeling. As with all other activities, its application is at the discretion of the master, its acceptance by the slave is expected.

Though the master may do things to make the discipline more bearable, for instance, by tying the slave up before he is beaten, it must be administered so as to have an effect. It is meant to be neither play nor fun. It's purpose is to modify behavior and redress wrongful actions or attitudes. It need not always be corporal: exile, prohibitions, chores, can all have the same effect.

Though the discipline can be imposed whenever the master desires, it really should be used as soon after the transgression as is feasible. The dread of an expected punishment can be difficult for a slave to handle, though some delay may be helpful in order to allow the slave to be punished by the dread.

A prolonged delay, though, will give an opportunity for the discipline to be forgotten, or at least for the severity of the transgression to fade. The slave will also see delay as hesitancy, indecision, apathy, or weakness on the part of the master. So apply discipline judiciously, promptly, and with confidence. Discipline is a master's duty, right, and friend.

There is more to the leather scene than play-acting. It can be more than pleasurable. Like all relationships, SM can provide an environment for personal growth and deep meaningful relationships. When two people come together with mutual respect and understanding, they open themselves to a world of miracles and delight. No matter what connotation you give to the word "rod," use it wisely and it will reward you immensely.

Chapter 30

THOSE TWO POINTS
OF PLEASURE

I can feel my tits today. They got a workout last night. My friend played with them, twisted and pinched them, and used clothespins as well. When the clothespins didn't hurt anymore, he took them off and used his fingers again. The pain was delightful. Somehow he knew I wanted him to do that.

This morning, he started in again. He went for my tits. There weren't any clothespins this time, just fingers and fingernails. He knows how to push the right buttons. Those two dark nipples are instant switches to turn me on.

It wasn't always that way . . .

Common wisdom—generally unspoken—is that sex comes naturally, and what you have and how you use it is what you're stuck with. There's no thought that sex can be taught or learned. Face it. We build our muscles and develop our minds. There are schools for dance, music, and architecture. There are gymnasiums and football camps, coaches, instructors, and teachers of all sorts. But we leave sex to be learned on the fly (so to speak), without any expert supervision, and the job is seldom done well.

Other cultures teach sex in various ways but we shy away from it. Sad to say, the majority of us learn it poorly, struggle with it often, and long for a better way.

I've always thought that my tits were just my tits,

useless since I am a male. I had no idea what they were for, and didn't think they would ever amount to much. I was wrong. The nipples on a man's chest can be the source of an immense amount of pleasure. That much I've learned.

A night in a bar where men expose their chests demonstrates that tits come in all shapes and sizes. What you don't see is that the variations can be developed. With playful attention, my own tits have grown in size and as they've done so, they've become a greater source of pleasure.

Leatherfolk call it TT—tit torture—a very deceptive title. I remember my first forays into tit work. Barely out in the leather scene, I'd put a clothespin on each nipple just to see what would happen. Invariably, I'd soon take them off. It was all pain. Well, almost all pain; hidden in the self torture was a heightened sense of arousal and a bit of pleasure.

With practice I could take the clothespins, and then tit clamps, for longer periods of time. And, with practice, the pain diminished and the pleasure increased. The idea that an aspect of sexuality can be developed, actually learned, is important. It points us to a way of being, a way of looking at things, that affords us greater possibilities.

Yes, we may think that we lack sensitivity in our chest. Yes, we may shun partners who squeeze our nipples, but the truth is that many of us can learn not just to tolerate such activity, but actually to enjoy it.

As I drove home from my friend's house, I could feel my tits rubbing against my shirt. I ached with a warm glow, both of pleasure and pain.

Playing with someone else's tits is another sensation. The pleasure is in the control, and in the giving of pleasure. I see my partner squirm, writhe, as I use his nipples to dominate him. With his two points of flesh between my fingers, I take control. He doesn't stop me. He has already submitted himself to my "handiwork." He knows that my fingers will bring him to his knees, bring him to surrender. I roll his tits between my fingers, feeling, pressing their flesh. I delight in the pain and pleasure on his face, his gentle, and not so gentle moans. He will do anything to convince me to stop, but hopes that I won't. I have him; he is mine.

Greg, an experienced bottom said, "They just don't understand what we gain when we submit to their domination."

There is more than control.

Bottoms have submitted, have hoped I'd pinch their tits for a reason. They want the pleasure I can give them.

The paradox is that we "sadists" enjoy inflicting pleasure. We give our submissives what they want: pain, confinement, humiliation, or domination. We make their nipples ache and feel good. That gift is a significant joy, a real turn on to a top. We do what we do for the pleasure we inflict. We enjoy, vicariously, the pleasure that our bottoms' tits are producing. We can only sense what's going on. But our senses tell us they're having one hell of a good time. We can tell by the glow on their faces, and the sighs in the their voices that they are having fun.

I don't know what makes it a turn on for me. I only know that a major reward to being a top is the knowledge that one's bottom is satisfied.

I could continue with ideas about sadism, or stories about tops who like to have their own tits played with. Instead let me just say that I hope your tits feel as good as mine.

Chapter 31

IT'S NOT THE CLOTHESPINS

Most leather scenes are playful and of relatively short duration. Physical pleasure is the sole measure of their intensity. They may contain aspects of emotional and psychological release, but these are short-lived and usually of a fairly superficial nature. At times though, there can be more to SM than a one-night stand or simply an orgasm and a good-night.

Most people don't think of clothespins as being part of a leather toy bag, but the truth is that they are often one of the first purchases a leather novice makes. Even the most advanced sadist keeps a supply of them handy.

Store bought tit clamps, alligator clips, and other such pinching toys are certainly prevalent, but clothespins retain a special place in one's collection of pleasure/pain devices. They are easy to acquire, inexpensive, cause no embarrassment when purchased, and need neither care nor significant investment. Where else can a person get 50 SM toys for under five dollars?

The simple wooden, spring type clothespins are a mainstay in my toy bag. They're easy to apply to various parts of a body and, although they inflict pain, they cause no permanent damage. They won't break the skin, permanently mark the tissue, or spread disease.

If you've never tried a clothespin on your nipple, I suggest you find one soon and simply apply it in the

149

privacy of your bedroom. I remember my first clothespin: it hurt. So I only left it on for a few minutes. The pain is one that generally builds as the skin under the clothespin is deprived of blood for longer periods of time. Eventually the area goes numb. The worst pain occurs when you take the clothespin off. When that happens the blood rushes back into the area and significant pain is felt for a moment. The sensations then turn into a kind of pleasure, depending upon one's tolerance, experience, and the amount of pressure applied by the clothespin.

I'll never forget the School of Lower Education held at the Mine Shaft in New York, sometime in the early eighties. It was my first exposure (I only watched!) to clothespins, and a lot of other SM as well. A master had his slave tied spread eagle to the wall. He then applied, in an attractive pattern, over 200 clothespins to the guy's chest, arms, thighs, and genitals. That blew my mind.

But as with many SM activities, there's more to clothespins than meets the eye.

On two different occasions, I had similar experiences with the application of clothespins. Let me illustrate my point.

I had been dating Steven for about ten weeks. Soon after we met, he asked me to be his master. I told him I was willing to start something between us, but since we were outside the Mercantile Exchange on the banks of the Chicago River, he'd have to wait for a more appropriate time and place.

We began dating seriously, and he soon won a place in my heart as my boy, and I got called a chicken hawk for the first time. I couldn't help it if Steven was a Daddy chaser! Anyway, I digress. Our scenes increased in intensity over the ensuing weeks. We grew fond of each other. He learned how to please and serve, which I expected. I taught him what he could endure and how to enjoy it. It was a mutually fulfilling time of training and affection. Steven was becoming a leatherman.

On the "night of the clothespins," he was kneeling buck naked next to my bed. His hands were tied behind his back. I looked into his eyes and over the next five minutes or so, I put twelve clothespins on his cock and ball sac, one by one. I don't remember what, if anything, we were talking about. I do remember being my typical demanding self. I wanted to take him a bit further tonight, past a limit, into new territory. There was an intense feeling between us, though I have to admit I wasn't reading the scene as well as I thought. He was taking everything surprisingly well. For a twenty-one year old novice he was doing fine. At least that's what I thought.

When I put on the twelfth clothespin, he lost his temper and told me to stop, to take the clothespins off. He didn't want anymore of this. Of course, I did as he asked. I ended the scene right then and there, but I wouldn't let him go home immediately. Instead. I convinced him to take a few minutes to talk things out. As we did, the real story came out.

It wasn't the clothespins that had set off his anger. Instead, in the pain and intensity of the moment he had flashed on images of his childhood. I was no longer a leathersex top. Instead, he saw his father, demanding perfection, pushing him to take it. It was an unpleasant experience, and one at which he had often and repeatedly rebelled. He didn't so much want to me to stop as he wanted the Dad of his childhood to stop. The clothespins and I had pushed him into an emotional and psychological area that was hidden and often suppressed. The scene was

151

a trigger for its release and revelation.

Experiences with depth, emotional release, and the gaining of insight are among the side-benefits of intense physical activity. Though we often forget, the various aspects of our life are intricately woven together. Emotion affects thought which affects body which affects action and reaction. Each side of us builds and feeds the others. Each "part" of us only seems to be a part. In reality we are one and complete in many dimensions.

I don't encourage anyone to make their leather scenes into therapy scenes. Such activity is best left to qualified counselors. But recognize that emotional and spontaneous reactions are possible and even probable. Don't be afraid of them, just relax and encourage your bottoms to do the same.

So if you think it's the clothespins, or the leather, or the kissing, remember it's not the clothespins. What is it? It's the life experiences that we bring to the moment, the fleeting experiences that add up to life.

Chapter 32

PAIN AND THE LEATHER LIFESTYLE

The leather scene is famous (notorious?) for its focus on paddling, whipping, cock, ball, and tit torture, and the infliction of pain in general. Because of that, how to handle the resulting pain is an often-asked question. The most obvious way, of course, is to avoid it. But avoiding pain denies us the satisfaction we're looking for. Pain holds a certain attraction, so we allow it into our lives.

Before I go too far (and some would say I went too far years ago!), I'd like to set some ground rules. I'm not writing about violence, harm, abuse, or coercion. They have no place in real SM activities. If any of these characteristics are present, then it's not what I'm into.

I'd like to take time as well to mention domestic violence. Coercion has no place in the life of leatherfolk. If consent isn't freely given, then it doesn't exist. Be careful of using or being abused by economic, emotional, or other subtle means of coercion. If you fear that you're in a wrong relationship, help is available.

Get yourself to a phone where you can talk freely and call any number of help lines that are available. Experts on domestic violence know how to help you and your partner. Remember we are talking about love, wherein there is no place for threats, fear, and coercion. Fortunately, the leather community knows the difference. We don't deny pain, but we do shun abuse.

Most people shy away from the possibility of being hit with a belt, or whacked with a paddle. Taking it a step further, few people want to have their body covered in clothespins, slaps, hot wax, or other uncomfortable SM devices. On the other hand, pain can be a rewarding experience, a door opening into a set of very positive feelings. In order for these "alternative" feelings to be felt, there are mental and physiological shifts to make.

Pain is pain, and pain hurts. SM pain is no different. When a loving master whips a trusting slave, wonderful things may take place, but the slave still feels the pain. He/she may not mind it or feel it for long. There may be cascades of pleasure, exceptional alternate sensations, deep mystical events, but there is pain. What is different is not that the pain ceases, but rather that we can change the pain into other kinds of feelings.

I once took part in a "Bun Warming Fund Raiser." I volunteered to allow the highest bidder to paddle my ass. As the high bidder was using the paddle on me, I felt pain. I have felt worse pain, since he certainly wasn't beating me unmercifully. I was leaning over a padded saw horse and thinking, "Well, this is a good show for the rest of the people watching. I hope we raise some good money for tonight's charity." What was foremost in my mind wasn't the pain, but the reason for the pain. I wasn't afraid of what was going to happen, so I remained fairly relaxed. In a very few minutes the paddling was over and my job was done. But the effect of the swats lasted. A half hour later, as I was standing at the bar drinking a beer, I noticed the warmth that the paddle had induced in my butt. My hand could actually feel the heat. It felt good. There was a certain satisfaction of having endured it as well as a feeling of pleasure. There was a slight euphoria in my body. The pain had been transmuted.

How is that done? There are various techniques. Physically, our bodies "defend" themselves from the trauma of pain by releasing endorphins into our system. These naturally occurring chemicals give us the slight euphoria that I experienced after my paddling. The more intense the pain, the greater the amount of endorphins released. This is similar to the effect of the "runner's high."

Mental techniques that can be used to tolerate or transmute pain include relaxation and focussing. The relaxation techniques include various forms of meditative and physiological exercises, such as breath regulation and muscle relaxation. Pain is intensified with the onslaught of fear and panic. Relaxation counters this natural tendency. Tensed muscles handle pain with much more difficulty than ones that are relaxed.

The other technique is to focus on thoughts and actions other than the pain itself. Just as I concentrated on the audience's pleasure and the funds being raised for charity, any distraction from the pain is helpful.

Many well trained bottoms, who are used to enduring pain, concentrate not on the pain they are receiving, but rather on the pleasure their top is receiving by administering it. I know that spanking turns me on significantly, and the boys I play with enjoy the fact that I am enjoying myself. They submit to it, not for the pain they endure but for the pleasure they create.

When I'm in the mood to redden a boy's butt, and there's a boy handy to do it with, I often have him lie with his face in my crotch and his arms around my waist. This position not only exposes his ass to my whip or paddle, but also gives him something to think about and to focus on.

It is just this kind of focus that will take a guy's mind off his pain, especially since most (gay male) bottoms are such avid cock-suckers!

Another technique, and one that works well in fantasy scenes is to gain satisfaction from knowing that you are able to withstand the pain. I know that it may not be PC to admit it, but I often withstand pain—but not injury—by thinking about the masculine character of "taking it like a man." Doing so makes me feel good about myself and my own strength. People may ridicule such thoughts but they are real for me and one of the reasons why I accept the paddling when it comes. In the end it proves something to me and that proof is satisfying.

We aren't into pain for the sake of pain as much as we see pain as a "doorway" into deeper and more meaningful experiences. These deeper moments are sporadic, somewhat unpredictable, and unfortunately, usually of a fleeting nature. But they still hold value and a significant part of SM's lure.

Chapter 33

FINDING A BOY

If I had fool-proof, complete-with-guarantee directions for finding one's boy, I think I'd make a fortune. That depends, of course, on whether or not the patent office would let me collect royalties on the process.

In Twentieth Century America one can't go out and buy a slave. The Emancipation Proclamation outlawed that practice. Purchasing sex is illegal for both vendor and client. Yentas are not easily found, though amateur match-makers seem to run about a dime a dozen. Even the time-honored tradition of marriage by parental arrangement (that's how my grandparents were hitched) has fallen into disrepute.

Alas, I have no easy answer. Now and again, I've thought I had succeeded in meeting and bedding the perfect boy (of legal age) only to find that our fantasies didn't complement each other as nearly as I or he liked.

Before I progress further, though, let me add a note about sexist language. I don't want to imply that one's boy has to be of the male gender. Let's just say that "boy," in this instance, is the generic name for the submissive of your dreams.

It's not always, nor need it be "man with man." I once met a very handsome, blond kid at a local bar, named "KB", the kind of young guy anyone would want to know. Cute, sparkling eyes, trim 'stache, impish look about him.

After we talked a while it became obvious that nothing would happen without Dad's permission. As it turned out "Dad" was a Lesbian. And KB was a lesbian with a pasted on mustache as well. She was out for a good time, exploring the masculine side of her life.

Another note is that when I write "boy" I mean "slave," though much of what is in this book applies to tops as well as masters, boys as well as slaves. Since most masters call their slaves "Boy" it's just natural for me to do so here. Isn't semantics fun? You get the idea, I'm sure. Whomever you want, you've got to find him or her, and that's not a quick and easy proposition.

I can give some ideas and some guidelines. In discussing this chapter idea with my friend, Lynn, I mentioned how impossible it was to find the right boy. Since he is looking for boy number three (slaves one and two happily under his control), he understood, but the smile on his face said, "Yes, it can be done." After all he had found Toby and Jim, hadn't he?

Lynn (who lives in Chicago) had been corresponding with an applicant named Terry from California. Terry's letters and photo looked promising. He called himself a total slave seeking complete domination. He wanted to start a new life under the absolute control of a man who would be his permanent master. He pledged no demand would go unanswered. He would bring no limits, no reservations. (Sounded hot to me!)

Lynn invited him to come for a mere weekend, offering, in fact, to help pay for the airfare. In reply, Terry declined, saying he wasn't ready for that kind of commitment. Put his name on the list of wanna-be's. I've had that experience time and time again: A boy faced with the possibility of turning a fantasy into reality, the reality

pales quickly and the fantasy becomes a "No, thank you."
There are enough master/slave relationships around to prove though that such states do exist. Finding the right boy takes patience and creativity. I also think it takes a large dose of openness. Don't hem yourself in with tight definitions about the right type either. After all, Mr. Perfect may not turn out to be Mr. Right. Mr. Right may never be what you thought you wanted, but you'll be much better off in spite of your preconceived ideas.

The way most guys talk, you would think that the "bar scene" is the most difficult and traumatic institution ever invented. The sentence "I hate bars" is an oft-repeated lament. But statistically, an awful lot of leatherfolk have met each other in bars, so that's not a bad place to start, or to continue, looking.

There are alternatives of course. In fact there are lot of ways to find that special person without ever venturing into a local gay drinking establishment. I've met lots of people in lots of different ways. You can do the same, if you're willing to make the effort.

I've lost count of the number of guys I've met through the modern day phenomenon of the computer bulletin boards. BBS'ing, as it's called, offers a low cost, right from your home, way to meet people. Of course, you've got to have access to a computer with a modem. That doesn't necessarily mean you have to own one though. I know several guys who log on to the BBS from work (not recommended, but if you can do it, more power to you), or from a friend's computer.

The classified ads work in the same way, though they are slower, since writing letters, and waiting for replies can take weeks or months. Do the ads get results? Well, I'm still friends with Gary, and we met more then ten years ago through an ad in *Drummer* magazine.

If you've never run an ad or answered one, just get yourself a PO Box and go for it. You'd also be advised to get a picture of yourself to send to the people to whom you write. Answering ads works just as well as taking out an ad. When I get in the mood to look that way, I'll send off a dozen or so form letters and then get more personal when the replies come back. I prefer to give my phone number and to talk over the phone, rather than relying on the mail.

Now, of course, there are talking personals. Instead of using the mail to answer ads, you can pick up the phone and leave voice mail. You'll get phone calls in response, not a bad first step toward meeting new friends.

There are also the 900 numbers. They work in much the same way as the computer does, but are invariably more expensive. When you talk to someone in whom you're interested, it's wise to get their number and call them directly, thereby reducing the per minute charges. A word to the wise here: be careful of your phone bill. The per-minute phone charges can run up quickly. The stories about $500 and $1,000 charges are true. You won't do that more than once, I'm sure.

Besides classified ads, magazines offer information about local and national clubs. But once again, you've got to make the first effort. These groups are often staffed by volunteers so at times their responses are a long time in coming. Don't give up, keep looking, and you'll find the friends you're looking for.

There is nothing wrong with being alone. In fact, there are times when solitude is both necessary and welcome. Loneliness, on the other hand, need not be a permanent condition.

You *can* find that boy. Doing so is just the beginning.

Once found you've got to take time to get to know each other, gain mutual trust, set limits, and agree on expectations.

I once had several marvelous months with a "boy." He was a handsome, cultured, attentive, and playful twenty-two year old. I taught him a lot about being my best boy and he responded wonderfully. He, though, had expectations that never crossed my mind. The relationship was doomed to failure from the start. The end of our relationship began when he couldn't consider the possibility of being only one of the slaves in my stable. He resisted me at that point, and I allowed him his opinion. From then on he tested me, finally refusing to call me "Sir." I punished him by exile from my bedroom for five days. That was the end. He thought the punishment too "wimpish." On his part, he had expected to be badly beaten in retaliation for his insubordination. In the end our expectations were too dissimilar and we went our separate ways.

I am no longer so quick to move into any committed relationship. Instead, I try to make it clear where I want to get, and that it takes time to know each other well enough to experience the intensity and depth that I seek. That doesn't, of course, mean that we don't explore possibilities on the way. Before I issue a list of rules I want to know where my "slave-applicant" is and where he wants to go. I will give most anyone the chance to apply, but I know that I need to be true to myself in what I do and with whom I relate.

For their part, even seasoned slaves need to be given time to learn how a new master wants to be served. It is here that the euphemism "training" becomes a real event. Teach your boy what you expect. If you only get what he wants, then you are no longer in charge. On the other hand, it is imperative that you grant the boy the right to speak, to question, and to learn. Boys have desires and dreams every bit as important as those of their masters. The challenge is to find a way to meet each person's fantasy without compromising the other's.

My newest "boy-in-training" likes to cuddle, wants to know my every move, and has a great need to feel accepted. He is just as starved (more so, maybe) for affection as for domination. I am willing to give him both. In fact, he will get affection in great measure. But for me to be comfortable in doing so, it must be at my discretion, my choosing. He's getting a furry master, but no teddy bear here!

What I would really like is my own live-in slave boy, one that fits the "best boy" description to a tee: an obedient masochist who can cook, clean, and do laundry. He should need little sleep but a lot of sex, and have enough of his own income that I don't have to support him. I'd like him to be more eager to serve, better built, and more intelligent than the usual Saturday night trick. That is what I really want. And I don't just want him for one night. I'd like to keep and enjoy him for a lot longer than that. I want him for life!

Even for those of us in the best circumstances (and that includes me), finding the right partner is no easy endeavor. On the surface I always advise (as above) that one use the shotgun approach. Try the bars *and* the classifieds *and* the computer bulletin boards. Let friends know you're looking. Join clubs, volunteer, be out-going and friendly.

But it's not as easy as all that. One summer, I answered almost 30 ads in *Drummer* magazine. From that I got twelve replies. I responded to all those who wrote me, and six sent return replies. I spoke with many of the men on the phone, with several I corresponded for three or four months. I actually got to meet three of them. One came to within a week of flying to Chicago to spend two weeks with me, but at the last minute fell in love with someone more geographically desirable.

I don't have any magic formula for helping that lover-to-be to knock on your door. I can't get that dream of mine either. The reality of the situation is that my life is full, incredibly happy, and I have more love in it than most people ever contemplate. So I'm not complaining. Those who know me well know that I'd better not complain either. Yet, that doesn't stop me from wanting a slave in my dungeon. I also want him in my bed, my kitchen, and my life! To have that happen, though, things have to change. And it isn't as if only he has to change to get here, but rather that I have to change to "get there" as well. Too often we think that it's the other guy or gal that keeps us from having the love we seek.

How do you find a slave? You let him find you and when he does, be what he's looking for.

Think of what you will be like when you have the boy you desire. How will your life be different? The critical question here is this: How do you have to change to be the person in the relationship you seek? What within you is keeping your future partner in the future? There are many reasons why that slave boy isn't here right now: I'm too busy, too intense, and have too many other relationships, few of which I'm willing to give up. I want him on my own terms and I'm not very willing to compromise. So I don't get what I want because a significant part of me probably doesn't want him.

After all, if I did, I would change enough to let him find

me.

Though it seems like another lifetime, there was a time that my income level was just too low and I wanted a more prosperous life. I spent years trying to find out what was wrong. It was only after I had worked through my fear of failure, my negative feelings about moving to another city, and my attachment to the comfort of the status quo, that I was able to make the changes that had to happen before I could find the job that would support me in the manner I wanted!

Chicago has been very good to me. I'm in the right place at the right time and I have the job I want. My income level has grown substantially. Additionally, I can get to the theater and the symphony with ease. I have a Great Lake to enjoy and beautiful Lincoln Park is only three blocks from my home. My family is well, my friends love me, and my writing appears in print every week.

What more can I ask for? Oh, my wants go on forever! And yes, I want a slave. Maybe we'll find each other, but if not let me say that that's all right, too.

I know the key to finding what I want is within myself. Look closely and lovingly at yourself and listen to your inner self as it tells how to find or be found by your "best boy."

Chapter 34

CONTRACTS AND COMMITMENTS

The attitudes held by both master and slave are what make their relationship work. That being the case, written documents describing how people will be a couple are merely external to the coupling itself.

Commitment, on the other hand, is intrinsically necessary. The simple fact is that you can't get into the serious beauty of SM without a committed partner. I'm not negating the fun, and sometimes the glory, of an SM scene between strangers, prostitutes and their clients, or people who just want to play "with no strings attached." But the best SM is with someone you know, trust, and with whom you have some kind of commitment.

I'll get to the ideas and experiences I've had with putting a slave under contract, if only because they make for interesting reading. But commitment is a much more important topic. That's partly because it carries a great deal of emotional baggage with it. Before we can really understand commitment, it needs to be debunked and defined to fit the freedom of a healthy leather scene.

I may be projecting when I write it, but the word commitment brings up connotations of "traditional" family values, including monogamy, fidelity, chastity, and morality. At the same time it makes us think about cheating, adultery, lying, and sneaking around. The reason for that is that we buy into the "Nelson Family Model" of husband, wife and two point five children living happily ever after. And there is nothing wrong with that model.

My parents have just celebrated 48 years of marriage, and I can easily assume that when my Mom says they've been faithful all those years, she's telling the truth. My parents aren't quite the Nelsons. My Dad used to leave home at 6:45 am to open the grocery store that supported us. He would return at 6 pm for a 15 minute dinner, return to work, and finally arrive home for the night at 10:30 pm. So much for family togetherness. It was survival. (If you heard me sing or play a guitar, you'd know that I'm not Ricky Nelson either.)

The commitment that I'm advocating is the only commitment that counts: "To thine own self be true." The operative words here are clarity, honesty, consistency. I'm talking about a relationship wherein each partner is able to find him or herself, express that self within the context of the relationship, and grow.

Leather is an arena for the radical. That means it allows for exploration and experimentation. It refuses to be pigeon-holed into some concrete category. Instead, it remains fluid, vital, and responsive. That doesn't mean, though, that its undependable. Every relationship must have some kind of stability. We need to care for our partners, and to be there "when it counts." If there is to be trust, there must be dependability. They go together.

Dependency gets a lot of bad press. We've turned it into an evil as dark as addiction. But face it: we are all addicts. Even the worst heroin user craves his regular hit of oxygen. The cleanest Republican still breathes. And yes, we need each other, and there's nothing wrong with that.

Suffice it to say that we ought to need each other,

depend upon each other, in a healthy way. If such isn't the case, then get out of the relationship as soon as you can, or get help to transform it into a healthy one.

Clarity: be clear about what you want in a relationship. Know yourself and your fantasies. Explore and experiment to see what you like and dislike. Let your play be a time to learn and, as you learn, use that knowledge to better define your goals and expectations.

Honesty: be honest with yourself about your desires and limitations. Don't kid yourself about what kind of relationship you're seeking, about what you're willing or unwilling to do. And, as difficult as it might be, share the clarity that you have with your partner honestly. Be willing to say "No." And be willing to live with the consequences of your honesty.

I know that I come down on the radical, idealistic side of the fence when I say it, but it's better to be without a relationship than to be in one that is dishonest.

Consistency: change is the only constant we really have. I'm not advocating stagnancy or a bull-headed stubbornness that refuses to change. What I'm suggesting is that you know yourself and stick to what you know about yourself. If you choose to be a master, be steadfast in your domination. Be consistent in your expectations, your demands, and your reactions. Expect the same from your slaves.

If neither of those options attract you, you can still be consistently versatile!

Having followed my advice (good luck!) you may want to give some kind of symbolic permanence to your relationship. This is where the contract comes in.

The first slave I ever had under contract was David, a man who lived in a neighboring state. We had been

167

corresponding for some six or seven months. He had
visited me in Indiana several times and was a wonderful
addition to my dungeon. That man knew (and probably still
does) how to serve, how to make me feel good. Our
relationship was intense and his letters to me reflected that
intensity. I incorporated some of the desires he had written
to me in the contract:

"i beg for assistance in controlling my actions and
handling my feelings . . . i want to be your slave and to
provide you with all the pleasure you want, any way you
want it . . . i need your domination, control and training to
be what you want me to be.

"When i am in your presence you have total control
over me as your slave . . . i am grateful for my master's
assistance in training, teaching, and disciplining me to be
a better slave for his pleasure . . . i want to kneel at your
feet and demonstrate that i am your submissive slave . . . i
want you to test my resolve and allow me to prove that i
am seriously your slave.

"i want to service your manhood . . . i look forward to
your using me for all your pleasure, and i am anxious to
smell and taste your master's cock, balls, and asshole. i
want to experience all of the endurance testing, discipline,
pain and humiliation you wish to give me . . . i wish to
prove that you own this hungry slave and that there are no
limits on ways i wish to bring you pleasure."

David was clear about what he wanted, and so was I. I
wanted David! So I wrote a contract that reflected our
desires, set attainable goals, made clear how he was to
obey me, and outlined my responsibilities as well. We
signed it one evening in my living room and sealed it with
drops of blood taken (safely) from each of our nipples.

The contract started this way:

"I hereby accept the submission of your person and your self to my mastery. By this instrument I agree to direct, train, and dominate you as I wish. Your servitude will continue for a period of twelve months, beginning on the day of the signing and sealing of this agreement, which will be on the day of your ritual dedication to me, that is June 11th, 1991.

"Your slavery may be renewed at my discretion.

"It is agreed that this period of slavery will be under my direction and control and will be subject to the following conditions."

The conditions I set included rules about how often we would communicate, i.e., "a minimum of once every two weeks via telephone in order to maintain my knowledge of your actions, guide my mastery of your life, and ascertain your progress. We will meet together for personal service to me at least once in every two months of the term of your slavery. I will determine the time and place of such meetings. Other, more frequent forms of communication, are encouraged."

I added requirements that determined the quality of his service to me: "We agree that fundamental to your slavery will be the practice of the virtues of trust, honesty, openness, loyalty, and obedience. Without the practice of these virtues in your relationship to me as master, there can be no true slavery. Their practice, therefore, is expected and required at all times."

I set goals for our relationship. These had been derived from his letters to me, and through our frequent discussions. They included being part of my "family" of slaves, "to further my development as master/lord over you and over others . . . to bring me physical, sexual, intellectual, emotional, and spiritual pleasure by the

169

submission and service of your self to my will . . . to be trained to do the above without failure, without rebellion, and without hesitation."

The contract also recognized some of the practical limits imposed by David's family situation and the distance he lived from me: "We acknowledge that this agreement binds us as master and slave dedicated to the accomplishment of our goals. This relationship will in no way prohibit the maintenance or development of relationships with others, except that for the duration of your slavery you will make the attainment of the goals herein described your first priority and the conduct of your slavery, in light of these goals, will take precedence, when such precedence is required, over other relationships, goals, and activities.

"You will restrict your sexual activity to me and to those to whom I assent, on an individual basis, to your having sexual activity.

"I recognize the preeminence of obligations to your family and career, and will prioritize your obligations to me in light of those obligations as well."

And lastly, I made clear that ownership was ownership. We were to be master and slave, not lovers, therefore the ownership, like any ownership was transferable:

"By your agreement to this document, you give me the right to transfer the duties, rights, and obligations of this agreement to any person at any time for the duration of this agreement. Those persons to whom I transfer these rights by gift, rental, or sale shall be deemed holding the rights of this agreement in my place and shall receive the same respect, service and obedience as due me."

Practically, David's slavery ended when I moved to Chicago and he wasn't able to see me with any regularity. By then I had another man "under contract." It was with him that the "transference" clause came into effect.

My slave Al met Vinnie at my house one weekend. They began dating and soon fell in love. Both Al and Vinnie were reluctant to tell me of their feelings, fearing that I would be angry.

I wasn't, since I realized that they really did love each other—and love is always grand! I gave Al to Vinnie as a gift, even signing Al's contract over to him. May not be legal, but it sure was romantic.

And that is really what we're all about: Not clinging or grabbing, but rather sharing, finding out who we are and living accordingly. It's just not a bad way to be.

Chapter 35

VERBAL ABUSE

As far as I can tell, communication is one of the most important of all human skills. Our ability to communicate seems to separate us from minerals, plants, and animals. I say "seems" because, for all we know, they communicate on their own terms just as well, perhaps better, than we do. We really don't communicate well at all. In spite of the written word, highly developed speech, electronic correspondence across miles, body language, and an innate ability for ESP, we often manage to misunderstand and to be misunderstood. And that's when we're only trying to get our message across. Imagine how the difficulties increase in the context of domination and submission, in the passion of a sexually charged dialogue.

Verbal abuse is a specific form of communication, and I'm not very good at it. Some folks get off on the idea of being called "shithead" or "rotten." Humiliation is an experience they strongly desire. Some masters enjoy the verbal put down of their slaves as unworthy, useless, stupid, etc. I'm not one of them. But, I do like to talk dirty. I like to use words for their shock value and, in so doing, defuse them and rob them of their negative effects. For instance, I like to call a cocksucker a "cocksucker" when he's sucking my cock. As Jiminy Crickett says, "It's factual, actual, everything is satisfactual."

I see verbal abuse as different.

If we go back to the goals of leathersex, we find ourselves reading that the first goal is empowerment. This entails encouragement, ego-building, and self-image enhancement. It calls for the positive affirmation of each partner.

It may be surprising to think, but empowerment doesn't only apply to the master. Slaves are meant to be empowered as well. In fact, it is this feeling of empowerment that, first surprises, then motivates many bottoms. Having endured the blows, the orders, and the submission to another, they discover their own strength. Understanding this makes domination easier, in so far as we masters enter into a creative, positive relationship, rather than a destructive, negative one.

Admittedly, I show the prejudices of my experiences and my world view. Some, in fact, have no trouble at all with verbally putting others down, and many bottoms enjoy the oral assault. It's not my cup of tea.

Verbal abuse entails a steady stream of name-calling, derogative orders, and a running commentary about what's going on in the scene. Since I prefer to accent the positive, such vocal activity is difficult for me. I prefer to see masters and slaves as equals in a complementary relationship. If the guy's an asshole, then why do I want him for a slave? Give me an intelligent, handsome, "ten" anytime.

I'm not alone in my low estimation of verbal abuse either. In his book, Ties That Bind, Guy Baldwin questions the healthiness of verbal abuse as well.

Enough said. If verbal abuse adds to your (plural) mutual pleasure, I will not condemn it, though I will question your motives and your clarity on the subject. Being the best master, I think, means that you care for

174

your slaves and help them to become the best slaves possible. They ought to be respectful, worshipful, and obedient, and it takes more than just an asshole to do that well.

Chapter 36

SO, WHAT ARE YOU INTO?

My mom says "Everyone to their own tastes, as Nelly kissed the cow." That does seem to be the case, especially in the leather community. We use all kinds of search techniques, symbols, and actions to realize, express, and experience our tastes. The more specialized one's taste, the more specialized the "signage" or the media. And yes, Virginia, there is a Santa Claus somewhere who will help you get just the kind of action you're looking for.

I don't consider myself a "fetish" kind of person, since my tastes run fairly middle of the leather road. I'm the more eclectic, "little bit of everything" kind of aficionado, but that really depends on your perspective. After all, some people consider leather itself, and here I mean the lifestyle not the fetish, to be a fetish.

Since you're reading this book for educational reasons (aren't you?), it's important to define our terms. My handy dictionary defines "fetish" in three ways, the third of which applies here: "something, such as a material, object, or often a nonsexual part of the body, that arouses or gratifies sexual desire." The list, of course, is quite extensive, including leather, piss, feces (called scat), feet, hair, sweat, tits and chests, piercings of all sorts and in all sorts of places on the body, boots, cigars and cigarettes, materials such as silk, spandex, and denim, underwear and/or jock straps, rubber and latex, both as toys and as clothing, and uniforms, especially military, law enforcement, and fire fighters. Now of course, I'm going to be in trouble because I'm sure to have left out someone's favorite fetish, so let me just conclude the list with "et cetera."

Not everyone is attracted to every fetish, of course. Take scat, for instance. One's desire to play in and with shit, the common term for scat, is a fetish. For reasons of health, custom, and taboo, it's not one often indulged in. But, believe me, when I say that there are some out there who find human excrement sexually exciting. Suffice it to say that ingestion of the substance is dangerous and should be avoided. Play safely, folks, I want you to be around to read my books for a long time.

But most fetishes, thankfully, are very safe. No one ever got a sexually transmitted disease by licking the top of a leather boot.

We often think of foot fetishes because foot and fetish are an alliteration. And feet are a popular turn on, though obsessive foot lickers and lovers aren't all that common. Having one's feet massaged with fingers, tongue, and mouth is exciting, especially if you are on the receiving end and the giver is a foot fetishist. (Use that word ten times and it's yours!)

There's a local leather bar, for instance, where a young man hangs out just for the pleasure of massaging the patron's feet. He is a foot fetishist.

It was at the same bar, by the way, that I recently met a man into leather as leather. When I went home with him, I was treated to the wonderful fulfillment of his leather fantasy. Though it loses something in the writing, he gave a moment by moment running commentary of the scene from his leather viewpoint. He asked me to put on a pair

178

of his leather high top boots and a motorcycle jacket. For his part he wore chaps, a cod piece, and a jacket. He knelt in front of me and asked me to "knight" him with a shiny leather motorcycle hat. We became lords of leather.

The scene moved to the bed where we kissed and licked in leather. This is where a "leather" scene really feels good. The scent of the cowhide fills your nostrils. The material helps build your body heat and you perspire. The smell of love-making mixes with the black armor we wear. And it's more than smell. The feel is sensuous, and then there is the sound. I love to hear leather against leather, rubbing, squeaking, speaking its magic vocabulary as we caress, push, lean into, and move on each other's body. Flesh inside of flesh rubs against flesh inside of another's flesh. Did I say magic? Maybe the first dictionary definition of fetish does apply: "An object that is super-stitiously believed to have magical powers, esp. of protection."

It was a hot scene and like the dictionary said, it aroused and gratified!

As I think about it, I might have a tit fetish. You've read my thoughts and experiences about tit play. I suppose that whether one considers nipples to be sexual organs or not determines if the love of tits qualifies as a fetish. Well, if he doesn't know already, tell Miriam Webster that tits are sexual organs. But then again, isn't all of our body sexual really?

Sorry, I digress. Back to fetishes.

I love to have my nipples worked over with clothes pins and clamps. When the clamps are stripped of their rubber padding and applied directly to the flesh, the pain can be excruciating, but fleeting, as it is transformed into pleasure. They hurt so good. I find that any attention paid to my tits is directly transferred to my genitals as excitement.

In fact, one of the fastest ways to bring anyone to orgasm is with the right kind of tit work. For those who know and whose tits are "practiced," the pleasure is immense. If that information leaves you cold, then let me assure you that pleasurable tit torture is an easily acquired taste. It's something that you can learn, and even teach yourself.

For some reason we consider fetishes to be dis-orderly, compulsive, and extreme. We dismiss them with comments like "Oh, that's a real fetish to her."

The uniform fetishists completely expose the falsity of that assumption. There is nothing more structured, considered, and exact then the mindset of the men and women of the American Uniform Association.

It is the mental association of uniforms with the values and characteristics of their wearers that is the turn on here. Uniforms prove that a great deal of what is sexual really takes place in the brain. When you fathom the reasons they love a person in uniform, you hit upon ideas such as strength, power, and authority. The uniforms represent these qualities. The mind links them to sex and brings on the gratification. When they say "It's all in your head," they know what they're talking about.

Knowing your desires and clearing away the mental noise that confuses that knowledge is what makes a fetish a turn on. But then, that is how anything works. The point here is to know yourself and your desires. Understand from whence they come, and if they are "true" to your inner self. Are they the real you?

Explore them, perhaps vicariously at first. Investigate their history, the organizations that promote them, their limitations, their "dialect." Meet the people who practice your dream fetish, and ask them to help you get started. Believe me when I say that there's only one thing that a fetishist loves more than talking about his or her fetish and that's to "do" it!

Chapter 37

I WENT TO THE OPERA INSTEAD

Three different friends invited me to Bob's party. They knew I'd be interested. After all, we writers need to keep up with the local social life, don't we? In fact, I had asked them to tell me about it and asked them if I could go.

Bob has a monthly "You're In" party. You pay five dollars at the door—that covers the cost of the beer you drink (I guess) and once inside you hand him your clothes, or at least the clothes you want to take off. The party itself is held in Bob's basement. Accouterments consist of a keg of beer and two (not one, but two) plastic kiddie pools. I don't think there's an official life guard on duty, but that doesn't matter. The guests aren't here to swim. They just want to shower. Golden shower, that is. You see, Bob hosts a monthly Piss Party.

I can see my editor squirming now. "You're not going to write about that!" he'll protest. But of course, in the interest of education, I'll do just that. My publisher will want me to state emphatically that some of the activities described in this chapter may not be safe and, therefore, YOU ought not to do them. In any case, ask your physician. Don't get sick because of something I wrote!

Piss scenes come in all varieties and as unhealthy as they may sound, can be quite safe. Safety, of course, means that the urine doesn't enter another's body orally, anally, or through the eyes or an open wound. Just pissing on someone won't harm them. On the other hand, make sure they're a willing participant or you may find yourself in deep trouble.

I first experienced a golden shower in New Orleans. I met this guy at *Jewel's*, one of my favorite bars in the French Quarter. In those days it was as raunchy as can be. Anyway, he took me home, and eventually took me into the bath tub, had me lay down, and aimed a warm, wet stream of piss at my naked crotch. The sensations were quite erotic to say the least, and produced an immediate orgasm.

In my years of leathersex, I've done my share of golden shower giving and receiving, but those scenes have been few and far between. Nevertheless, there are those for whom golden showers hold a strong attraction. What that attraction means and how it is practiced varies widely.

For most, piss scenes involve pissing on a person or being pissed on. It's really as simple as that. Others take it a "step" further, and drink piss, usually "from the tap" but occasionally in other ways. For others it may involve "wetting one's pants" or playing with diapers. In any case the meaning of such activity is hard to explain.

For some it represents a "manly" sharing, for others it is a form of submission, domination, or humiliation. Some (a minority) see it in terms of genital worship. Remarkably, some like the taste, the idea, or just the thrill.

If you've read this far and aren't totally disgusted, I might point out that it's really not as bad as it sounds and given certain situations it can be a very erotic experience.

Of course, the experience varies widely, as the smell of urine and its taste is highly individualized. In an attempt to educate, suffice it to say that "morning piss" is quite strong and really hard to drink, while urine produced from a sufficiently large intake of beer has a high water content and is quite dilute in taste. Other than that you'll have to get your information first hand, so to speak.

To spare you one difficulty though, I will share a quick bit of trivia. In the interest of self education (read "to satisfy my curiosity"), I tried to drink a glass of my own urine several years ago. I was home alone (shall we make a movie of it?) and thought I'd see what it was like. Unfortunately, I had forgotten that I'd been taking these awful tasting pills for about a week. Well, if I thought they were ugly tasting in pill form, let me assure you they were horrendous when they came out in liquid form. So much for that night's experiment!

Actually, I prefer to do such things in quiet intimate ways with people I really like. I'm talking about a level of intimacy that goes way beyond one night stands and quick tricks. Not everyone feels that way of course. Most people follow our culture's mores. For them, urinating is dirty, disgusting, and an obligatorily private—therefore—solo activity.

I understand that some cultures see it differently, even to the point of ingesting a certain amount of urine for what they believe are reasons of good health.

I guess that a bit of piss now and then never really hurt anyone, but those whose immune systems are compromised ought to avoid drinking it, not that the rest of us ought to make a steady diet of it.

The guys who meet monthly at Bob's "You're In" party see it differently than most. Without putting words in their mouths I'd guess they enjoy the intimacy of it, the manly odor, the iconoclasm that it represents. It does seem to go back to the primal urge I wrote about in Chapter

Seventeen, "The Thin Layer of Civilization."

One of these months I'll have to drop in at Bob's and see what his guests are doing. I never did make it to the party. I know it does my reputation no good, but I went to the opera instead. Just proves that we leatherfolk are widely diverse in our tastes. I guess Bob's guests prove that as much as I do.

Chapter 38

FUCKING

I suppose that for sensibility's sake I ought to come up with a better title for this chapter. But as I sit here typing, I can't. You see, not only do I like the activity of fucking, I like the word. I like it for its shock value, for the way it flies in the faces of those who want to sanitize, legitimatize, and civilize the wonderfully basic and primal event called sexual intercourse.

The word "fuck" is common enough today to appear in my dictionary. It is noted as "obscene," its origin unknown. Someone once told me that it was an abbreviation of "for unlawful carnal knowledge." I don't know if it is or not, since no one has ever taught me anything about fucking, or sexual intercourse for that matter.

My parents didn't, neither did the priest who explained (if that's what you called it) sex to me and the other boys in my eighth grade class. My friend Jack borrowed a book on sex from the library when we were high school sophomores, but, other than the sketchy paragraph in there, instructions were nonexistent.

I was well into my own coming-out process when I first fucked my friend Mike. At the time he was a trick I had picked up at a local bar. I remember him wanting to be fucked early that Sunday morning. I obliged, and was astounded to see that he really liked having a cock (my cock) up his ass. I, of course, didn't try the same feat with my anus until a good three years later. And yes, it hurt the first time. And yes, sometimes it still hurts.

Those of you who still think that leather is about clothing, ought to know that leather is also about fucking. Of course, it's about a lot of other things as well. And there are a large number of ways to have great leather scene and still not fuck. In the age of AIDS, that's no wonder, I'm sure. But if you see leather as striving toward ecstacy and bonding, then chances are you're going to be part of a scene where a finger, cock, prick, dick, or penis (choose one) is inserted into an ass, anus, vagina, pussy, or cunt (choose one).

No one ever (except *in utero*) comes as close to another person as when he (or she) is inside the other, or conversely as when he or she has the other person inside them. The receptive part can squeeze and caress the inserted member. For its part the inserter can stroke and poke the insertee in wonderfully sensuous ways. The result is pleasure.

For the top, the pleasure often leads to orgasm. Surprisingly, many bottoms don't come when being fucked, but do get significant enjoyment and satisfaction in the activity. For those comfortable and knowledgeable in the techniques of love-making (another euphemism for fucking), orgasm remains the end (as in purpose) of sex but the act of sex is widely regarded as much greater than the orgasm itself. In fact, for many leatherfolk, orgasm is overshadowed by all the pleasures derived before orgasm.

In light of AIDS, many partners refrain from orgasm during fucking. Even though they go at it with a high margin of safety by using condoms and a virucidal lubricant, they withdraw prior to orgasm and have their ejaculation outside of their partner's body.

The whole point of fucking is, after all, intimacy and we should be and can be creative in ways to accomplish that goal. The physical inclusion of one's member in another's body is only one way that fucking accomplishes its objective. The bonds of unity in SM fucking (i.e., safe, sane, and consensual) are formed with one's emotions as well as one's flesh and blood.

We in the Western World don't often consider the energies of our ethereal bodies. Those of the East, particularly those who practice Yoga, Tantra, or any of those related Buddhist, Vedic, and Hindu Philosophies, have much to teach us in this area. Suffice it to say that there is more to fucking than just fucking. What has always attracted me to leather is the willingness of its adherents to explore, experiment, and actually devote time, energy, and thought to sex and sexual pleasure.

I'm not advocating the quick fuck that turns a trick into an object, a "fucker" into no more than a human dildo, though there are certainly enough reasons to have a quickie now and again. In the early days of several of my relationships it was not uncommon to do it on the couch during a half hour lunch break. But serious fucking, like anything else worth doing, takes time. Develop your technique, prepare the space, go at it slowly, build to climax. The operative word here is "slowly." Make fucking playful, while keeping it deliberate and varied. I was going to add the word tender, then thought about fucking being rough, and finally realized that the best word is varied, since both tender and rough have their places in intimacy.

There are times for ramming one's rod, and for riding an erect cock as if it were a wildly rocking horse, but the

189

best fucks are crafted with a gradual rise toward climax. Some even advocate that one develop the ability to have an orgasm without ejaculation so that multiple orgasms become possible in a shorter period of time.

Our culture has a fundamental prejudice against sex. I've railed enough against that premise already. Americans, and probably most of the societies on this planet, are embarrassed and ashamed about fucking. Hence, the lack of available instruction (not to mention unwanted pregnancies and sexual dysfunction).

I mentioned to a friend that I was writing about fucking and he said "Why? What's to learn?" It has to be written about because attitudes about sex as "being private" and "being dirty" are our misguided heritage. We choose to pretend that satisfactory sex is merely instinctual, needs no prompting, and is best gotten over with as soon as possible. In my adolescence, intercourse was discussed in terms of "marital obligations, procreation, and the alleviation of concupiscence." Those are hardly terms that engender pleasure. Fucking is about pleasure. Make that pleasure with care, responsibility, and intimacy. Make it safe fucking, and make it fun. Learn how to fuck—and how to get fucked. Read, watch, discuss. Approach fucking as a blessing. The world will be a better place if we do.

Chapter 39

SO, YOU'RE A TOP

I'm the first to admit that definitions do no more than help us communicate with each other. They are of little value in establishing relationships. Yes, they help us understand relationships, but in the passion of relating they quickly fall by the wayside. Relationships are defined not by some abstract terms about roles and stereotypes, but rather by the two people in the relationship itself.

Versatility certainly has a lot to say for itself. I'm a firm believer that anyone can be top or bottom. It all depends upon with whom they find themselves relating. On the other hand, consistency has a lot to say for itself, and there certainly are tops and bottoms who seldom deviate from their chosen roles.

But more often than not, the appearance of topping or bottoming is just that. Now you've got to read that line in the context from whence it comes. As you probably can tell by now, I take my leather seriously and look to have serious master/slave relationships. But what I expect and hope for is not what one might call the norm, even in leather society. Most people, for a wide variety of reasons, not all of which are wrong reasons, don't venture into the level of intensity and commitment that I've been exploring and writing about.

And that's OK. Once again, you have to define your relationship as you and your partner wish it to be. You certainly may want it to be other than the ones I've defined in these pages, and in my life.

On the other hand, there is some importance to honestly naming a situation for what it is. The most satisfactory relationships have clarity and honesty as their hallmarks. Be careful not to coast along on appearances. In due time, your bubble will burst, and you'll end the relationship scratching your head, wondering what went wrong and why you didn't really get what you wanted.

To be more specific about the master/slave scenario I've been proposing, you'll find that very often SM activities seem to be one form of domination, when in fact they are another. If you haven't experienced that yet, then let me say it this way: in many situations, the top is the bottom and the bottom remains firmly in control.

I once interviewed (over the phone) a man who wanted desperately to find someone to take control of his life, at least on a part time basis. This man thought I was the perfect leather master, the one whom he could finally trust and to whom he could surrender. During the several phone conversations we had, it was obvious that this 55 year old professional was just starting out on the leather path. As we talked about experiences and expectations, he volunteered that he really wanted to be fucked. At his age that was an event still waiting to happen. No problem, you think? Well, that's true. After all it is certainly a master's prerogative to fuck his slaves.

The problem (quickly dispensed with I might add) was that this wanna-be slave went on to tell me how to fuck him. In that instance he assumed control of the relationship, directed me according to his desires, and turned me into a his slave, one who would be doing the fucking, but a slave no less.

I've experienced this phenomena over and over again, especially with my friends who like to get fisted. I remember a night in San Francisco, many years ago and pre-AIDS, when I fisted a guy. An hour after we started, I had been reduced to lying prone on the bed, my arm in the air as he slid up and down my wrist and fist. I didn't feel like a top, I felt like a dildo.

So, you want to be a master? Then be careful to master. Many bottoms, of course, don't want to be slaves. They aren't willing to surrender themselves to anyone. You'll find yourself playing with a lot of men and women like that, and we must respect their decisions to maintain control. But who are you and what are your goals? There comes a time in a master's development that he or she has to say "I won't be your slave any longer." Rather than abandon your desire to control in order to satisfy the fantasies of a bottom, begin to find men and women willing to share the kind of relationship you seek. That's not an easy task, but if you approach it seriously and honestly, it can happen.

I've found that to make it happen there needs to be a careful pace and a clear direction. Don't rush into commitments and agreements. Remember that for the two of you to find what you seek, there needs to mutual understanding and trust. Masters and slaves don't become so to each other immediately. Instead they grow in commitment and mutual faith over time. The way to do that is to be clear about what you want and to communicate that to your partner. Until you are clear that you intend to master and that you will eventually take authority and responsibility for the relationship, you won't be able to assert yourself as you think you'd like. Instead, you will find yourself continually fighting against a bottom whose goals may not complement yours.

I'm not saying that you are going to be in control completely at the onset of the relationship. In fact, chances are high that in many ways you won't ever be in complete control. After all, even the most avid masters enjoy having their slaves do the chauffeuring and that puts them in charge of the car! And I'm not putting down pushy bottoms. In fact, they are the successful ones, because they know what they want and they've found ways to get it.

What I'm saying actually is for you to act the same way. Know what you want and live your life so that you can get it. Reconcile whatever ambivalence you feel, accept your ability and right to control, and make it clear to your partners that that's what you really want.

Go for it. The world, and not just the leather world, needs more people willing to lead, to direct, and to take control of their own lives. Believe me, many of those bottoms out there really *are* waiting to find a master. It's just that that's such a damn near impossible thing to do.

Chapter 40

WHAT DO WE DO NEXT?

Saturday night at AA Meat Market is one of those standing room only nights. The back bar, its lighting dimmed, its music loud, can be packed shoulder to shoulder with leathermen in their great variety of dress and undress. AA's back bar has a dress code. In order to enter you wear a "major" piece of leather (chaps, vest, or jacket), a uniform of some kind (police, army, etc.), or go shirtless.

As the night lengthens into early morning, the feelings in the room get increasingly intense. The video screen casts the sight of porno stars doing "leathersex" through the smoke filled atmosphere. In the far corners, men fondle and kiss. Some may be lovers, but not a few have just met and are conducting their weekly "find a partner for the night" ritual. Most men are content to stand and watch, glancing from the video to someone across the bar. They circle the room and leave it for the less crowded front areas. They may watch a game of pool or check out who's sitting at the front bar. They chat with friends. It's a usual procedure—just call it cruising.

The onslaught of AIDS has certainly changed the extent of promiscuity and casual sex. What goes on these days is far removed from the permissiveness of the time between Stonewall and HIV. No doubt, anonymous sexual encounters still occur. Nevertheless, we're generally more careful, more hesitant to rush into sex, and more willing to play safely. There's more mutual "jack-off" activity and less shared raunch and unprotected "take it up the ass" sexuality.

On the face of it, the focus of cruising is sexual release: mere hedonism, thrill-seeking, and attention-getting. But appearances are deceiving. I am not naive enough to believe that those appearances are completely false. We are propelled by a wide variety of motives, commendable or not. Basic motives of sex and quick gratification are prevalent in our disposable, microwave culture. But to dismiss cruising as looking for "flash in the pan gratification" is to miss underlying human needs. Beneath the leather, the posing, and the S&M ("standing and modeling") is a real search for bonding. Like everyone else, leatherfolk want to know they are part of a community. Saturday night rites are the externals of a quest for belonging. We desire to be in union with our own kind, human kind.

I'll grant that the trappings of rope, chain, leather, and other fetishes are alien to the middle class "family value" crowd that wants to pass as "normal" and relegate us to being "sick." Nevertheless, the leathers are coverings that adorn a precious human nature. More bluntly: they clothe human souls. I'm neither exaggerating nor projecting when I say that the back bars are filled with warm, caring, and often lonely people. Though they may settle for the quick blowjob or one night stand, the preference, as masked as it may be, is for family.

Of course, each of us defines family differently. My dream family isn't the usual two and one-half children in the suburbs. It is unique to me. Likewise, you deserve your own "home and hearth," replete with the "kin" you desire.

Give me half a dozen hunky, honest, open men, free of guilt and shame. Men whom I can trust, who will listen and respond. I'd like a good fuck now and again, but what really matters is the relationship. My family will be comfortable whether clad in leather, buck naked, or dressed for the symphony. We'll share the rent and dishes. Each will have a rightful place at the table. Masters will rule; slaves will serve. The only acceptable limits will be our own potential. We'll be true to our inner selves, and honor the inner selves within each other. To expect perfect harmony is unrealistic, but we will face disagreements with mutual respect and crises with love. For families are for growth and challenge as well as solace and comfort.

I cruise. I'm apt to move between the front bar and the back as often as (more often than?) most. I've had my share of one night stands and quick self-gratifying sex. But I recognize such pastimes as fleeting. The ropes and cuffs have to come off in the morning, but the bonds of love stretch as far as two people can roam.

That's what I think the future is all about. Creating sustainable and nurturing relationships is what leather is really about. It is where leather is "going next." It's been the same since the days of motorcycle clubs, the Gold Coast, and when the "Old Guard" was still young.

Where do we go from here? The goals listed in chapter six still apply: Empowerment, Ecstacy, and Bonding. Though the great prophets may have put it differently, the best of these is bonding. That is both the present and the future of leathersex.

I trust your future will be filled with the partners and the experiences you seek. Have fun, and love each other, in and out of your leathers.

ABOUT THE AUTHOR

Simply put, Jack Rinella is a free-lance writer who writes for several regional and national publications. He brings over ten years' experience in the leather world to his writing, but a listing of what he's done goes far beyond the confines of a dungeon.

Born in upstate New York of Italian-American parents, Jack has been a high school and college teacher, a drug rehabilitation counselor, a cook, a salesman, a Catholic seminarian, a Pentecostal minister, an advertising copy writer, and a graphic designer. He's done stints at printing, publishing, telemarketing, head-hunting, and computer consulting.

He now lives on the North side of Chicago where he passes the time writing, cruising, and falling in love, whenever he can.

Looking For More Sexuality Books?

We publish and sell a variety of great non-fiction and fiction sexuality books and publications. To receive a catalog and mail order information write to:

Daedalus Publishing Company
584 Castro Street, Suite 518
San Francisco, CA 94114-2578 USA

or send email to:

daedalus@bannon.com

or send a fax to:

(415) 487-1137

or visit our web site at:

http://www.bannon.com/daedalus